SCIENCE
OF
BREATH

SCIENCE
OF
BREATH
A Practical Guide

Swami Rama
Rudolph Ballentine, M.D.
Alan Hymes, M.D.

Published by

The Himalayan International Institute
of Yoga Science and Philosophy
Honesdale, Pennsylvania

© 1979 by The Himalayan International Institute
of Yoga Science and Philosophy of the U.S.A.
RR 1, Box 400
Honesdale, Pennsylvania 18431

04 03 02 01 00 99 98 97   13 12 11 10

The paper used in this publication meets the minimum requirements
of American National Standard for Information Sciences—Perma-
nence of Paper for Printed Library Materials, ANSI Z39.48-1984.

Library of Congress Catalog Card Number: 79-65517

ISBN 0-89389-057-X

Contents

Acknowledgments

The authors would like to express their thanks to Edwin Funk, M.D. for his valuable technical advice, John Miller and Anne Craig for their help in preparing the manuscript and Dave Ballew for the artwork. Their labors have not gone unappreciated.

Foreword

This book is an examination of the breath—how it integrates different levels of man's being into a functional whole, what the nature of the interactions occurring on various levels is, and it includes practical methods for modifying these interactions. The scope of discussion is vast, ranging from the physical movements of chest and abdomen to the functioning of internal organs and the molecular reactions of respiration as well as to the subtle play of energy flow and its interaction with the mind. Precisely because its ripples touch upon so many human functions, a thorough understanding of the breath provides a powerful tool for expanding one's awareness of the various dimensions of body and mind as well as for use as a therapeutic modality.

The importance of the breath can be better appreciated by observing some of the mind's properties, for the mind tends to assume that apparently constant, or slowly changing features of the environment, or body are in actuality constant. It therefore filters many of these events out of conscious awareness in order to avoid a confusing barrage of sensations. This allows it to focus on the more significant changes which may relate to survival or other basic needs. In other words, a new pattern of thought or a new activity initially attracts much conscious attention, but with frequent repetition it be- comes unconscious and habitual. For example, walking is effortless for any adult; it occurs on an unconscious level and requires little or no conscious attention (although the conscious mind can easily intervene if necessary). However, the process of integrating the movements of walking into the mind took place only after years of trial and error throughout childhood. Only then did it become a habit and operate effectively on an unconscious level.

The internal organs (e.g., heart, kidney, liver) respond in a similar manner. Biofeedback research has shown that some of the physiological activities of these organs, previously labeled involuntary, can be conscious- ly controlled with training. In most people, however, this activity is unconscious, and much practice is necessary in order to be proficient in its conscious control. This is in contrast to the voluntary muscles which are more easily controlled on a conscious level.

Breathing is unique as a physiological function, as it lies midway between the internal organs and the voluntary muscles, insofar as the ease with which it can be consciously controlled is concerned. For example, depending upon one's proficiency in dealing with the breath, the rate and depth of breathing can be altered, but involuntary reflex activity limits the degree to which this can occur. These reflexes act as safeguards to pre- vent overextension of one's capacity. They are especially important in connection with breathing, since the flow of breath is essential to life, and the need to breathe is one of the most fundamental survival instincts. This in part reflects the key role played by oxygen in metabolism (or the process of supplying energy to the body), for without oxygen the body cannot convert food into usable energy.

Modern science has come to understand many of the principles involved in the physical aspect of breathing, from the muscles and organs which transport oxygen into and throughout the body down to the molecular reactions of metabolism. However, the purely intellectual appeal of these complex physiological systems has limited the scientific community's concept of the breath to the physical level only, even though the most casual reflection indicates that the significance of breath extends beyond its purely metabolic functions. For example, one's own personal experience suggests that there is a relationship between emotions and the breath, for most emotional states, especially if they are intense, appear to be associated with changes in breathing. The sob of grief and the trembling breath of anger are common examples which reflect this interconnection. In addition, physical stimuli such as pain and exercise can act to change both the breath and the emotional state.

Once these observations are studied a whole series of questions arises: What is the nature of the relationship between emotions and body and breath? What is the underlying vehicle? Does the breath interact with other realms of mind? Can emotional and physical states be altered by changing the breathing patterns?

These are some of the questions to which *Science of Breath* addresses itself. Each chapter develops one aspect of the central thesis that the breath is the link

between body and mind, and the authors weave together
the diverse scientific discoveries of the West and the rich
experiential insights of the East into a thorough and
balanced exposition. After the basic tenets of the book
are outlined in an extensive introduction, Dr. Hymes
presents the physiology and anatomy of the lower respiratory tract from an unusual perspective and examines
the physiological and psychological effects of various
breathing habits. A discussion of the nose (an oft-maligned
but rarely understood organ), and the upper respiratory tract follows in a chapter by Dr. Ballentine. Here,
this portal into the body is examined in terms of the
preparatory functions it exerts upon the incoming air-
stream and the complex patterns of nervous activity
and energy flow which this evokes. In the final chapter
Swami Rama describes the vehicle for the body-mind
interface: *prana*. According to the ancient yogic texts,
prana is the most subtle unit of energy, and here the
author discusses its organization into a *pranic* sheath,
or energy field, which underlies the physical structure
and functioning of the body and which is potentially
under the control of the mind.

But the goal of *Science of Breath* is to present
theoretical knowledge regarding the breath in such a
way that it can be applied as a tool for personal growth.
To this end a series of practical exercises and techniques
for systematically working with the breath and controlling the flow of *prana* is described in detail. These serve
to expand one's breath awareness, for as one observes
the way in which one uses his breath, various unconscious breathing habits are identified, and replaced with

more beneficial ones. Just as a child overcomes his clumsiness by becoming aware of his body and learning to walk, so does breath awareness gradually free the mind from relating to the breath on an unconscious level, and this brings it under greater conscious control.

As the link between body and mind, breath can intervene in the activities of either level. With an increased awareness and control of the subtle aspects of breathing, these interventions can effect deep physical and psychological changes. *Science of Breath*, then, opens up new avenues of being to the conscious mind, providing a powerful tool in the pursuit of truly holistic health and personal growth.

John Clarke, M.D.
Honesdale, Pennsylvania
May 25, 1979

One

Why Breath?

Many will be surprised to see a whole book devoted to the subject of breathing, for the study of breath has not received very much attention in Western medicine and physiology. In a letter to the editor printed in a recent well-known medical journal, a practicing physician was complaining about the time and money wasted on research in trivial areas of study. "The next thing you know," he lamented, "someone will be writing a book-length dissertation on 'How to Breathe'!" He could not imagine a subject more trifling or a process more obvious than that of breathing. Of course breathing is a vital process. If you don't breathe, you don't live, so everyone will agree that it is important in that sense. Yet most of us would say, "Either you're breathing or you're not breathing. If you're breathing, everything is all right. If you're not breathing, then obviously you'll die. It's that simple, isn't it?"

Perhaps it's not that simple at all. In the Eastern traditions there have long been those who would spend decades studying the breath. In fact, there are entire monasteries where most of the work centers around the study of breathing, and it is said that many of the so-called "feats" performed by yogis are managed primarily on the basis of a control of the breath. But why would such emphasis and importance be placed on an ordinary, everyday process like breathing?

The Mind/Body Problem:

Our difficulty in understanding why breathing might be so strategic stems in part from our Western way of looking at the world and the philosophy on which this is founded. In the West our way of understanding our universe is based primarily on the study of material phenomena. We take solid things and analyze them physically and chemically, and as a result we gain some understanding of that aspect of their existence. Our laboratory science is based on the manipulation of matter and its measurement. Our physicians are accomplished in anatomy and physiology. Our philosophical stance is basically a materialistic one.

In a similar way, our approach to understanding the human being is also primarily physical. Our scientific study of man is based essentially on the study of his body, the part we can touch, that which is tangible, measurable, and which can be examined under the microscope. The scientific studies that we trust and feel most comfortable with are those which treat what is objectively observable and material. When our research strays from this world of material objects and begins to attempt the study of other phenomena, we begin to feel a bit less sure of ourselves, and the question inevitably arises, "Is this really scientific?"

These doubts about the scientific validity of nonphysical studies are especially evident with respect to research in psychology, yet the mind is obviously another very real level of our existence—one with which we cannot avoid coming to terms, but one which is nonphysical.

The twentieth century Westerner's interest in the mind is equaled only by his uncertainty as to how to approach it. It can't be felt, tapped, dissected or measured. It can't be put on slides and viewed under the microscope. It can't be tested with electronic instruments. Yet our subjective experience assures us that there is such a thing as the mind and that it is very important. We are all aware of our thoughts; we are aware of thinking. We are aware that something is going on inside, and we admit, however grudgingly, that the workings of the mind are in some way behind most of what we do with our physical bodies and usually determine the way in which we manipulate the physical world.

Yet in the West we remain very confused about the relationship between the mind, or mental, realm and the tangible, measurable, physical world. How does the physical body relate to the mind, and what is their functional interaction? This is more than a mere theoretical or philosophical question. The problem of mind/body interaction is one that plagues our medical scientists and baffles our psychologists. When the physician fails to alter the physical body to the patient's satisfaction, he throws up his hands and says the problem must be "mental." When the psychologist is unable to help the patient reorganize his mental world, he shrugs and says, "Perhaps you should see a medical doctor to make sure there's not some physical problem here." Countless patients shuttle back and forth between frustrated psychotherapists and puzzled physicians while the psychosomatic specialist, the person who would understand the integration of mind and body, is yet to appear solidly on the scene.

How do the two connect, the mind and the body? How are they related? Our Western science seems to have run into a dead end on the question. But the philosophy of the East, especially that out of which the science of yoga grew, offers a context within which some answers may emerge, for yoga includes the study of both the body and the mind—both the physical and mental realms. But it includes much more than that; these two levels of functioning, the mental and the physical, are only a small part of the total spectrum of phenomena encompassed in the study of yoga.

Since ancient times yoga masters have spent many long hours going within themselves, studying and trying to unravel the connections existing between their various levels of existence. They have discovered that, besides the physical body and the mind, there are higher levels of functioning that are also important. For instance, they have uncovered and explored something beyond thoughts, a consciousness they have described as a "nonthinking" level of heightened and broadened awareness that could only be approached by stepping outside the arena of thoughts. This process of inward attention that allows one to explore this level of consciousness has come to be called, *meditation.*

Meditation is a technique used to deal with those levels of functioning operating beyond the mind, those levels we might call "higher consciousness." This is one aspect of yoga, this process called meditation. It is not, however, the only aspect of yoga which also includes physical postures *(asanas)* which have to do with learning to control, regulate and be aware of the physical level.

Then there are practices that have to do with the manipulation and regulation of the purely mental functions—concentration, for instance. Yoga is based, then, on understanding the human as a multileveled being, one with a series of distinct levels of existence—the physical, the mental and what lies beyond the mind.

But in our discussion so far we have omitted mention of another, and very important level: This is a level of existence, or a level of functioning, that links and lies between the mind and the body, for according to the teachings of yoga the mind and the body do not directly interact. Rather, they relate to each other by way of an intermediate level of functioning which lies between them. The indifference of Western science to the possibility of such an intermediate level is perhaps why the relationship between body and mind is so obscure. This is perhaps why we have remained stuck with a "mind-body dualism" which seems to split our science of man asunder, leaving it in two separate and irreconcilable camps: that of the psychologist, or humanist, and that of the physical scientist and laboratory researcher.

The "hard-nosed" scientist is sure that anything worthy of study is physical and material. If he wishes to deal with man's actions and behavior he limits himself to studying and measuring the movements of the body, the production of speech or the test performance of an individual. He may think of himself as a psychologist, but he prefers to label himself, "behavioral scientist." The mind itself he dismisses, convinced that it is not amenable to study. This seems to be a trend of the times, related perhaps to the increasingly materialistic orientation of our culture. In the last century, by contrast, the "idealist" went to the other extreme, dismissing the validity of the physical world and claiming that all which exists is mental. Fortunately in the East, and in particular among the Himalayan practitioners of meditation, the relationship between body and mind has been explored and found to constitute a distinct and important entity in itself, one which harmoniously occupies an appropriate place in the whole spectrum of existence, from the physical up to the higher states of consciousness. According to the ancient teachings, the intermediate level of existence that relates the body and the mind is separate and "real." It has its own properties, its own nature and its own topography. Moreover, it is explicitly taught that this intermediate level has to do primarily with energy.

The Multi-leveled Nature of Man:
    The progress of Western science has pushed us, slowly but surely, closer to this point of view. We have found it increasingly impossible to study the physical without beginning to become aware of a level of phenomena that is non-physical, which we here call "energy." In fact, we cannot study the body without becoming aware that it functions on the basis of energy. We end our study of anatomy by becoming interested in physiology. We end our study of physiology by beginning to deal with electrical phenomena. Physiology is based on movement, action, and the functioning of the organism. Such functioning always involves energy.
    The Newtonian physicist was interested only in mechanics. He was interested primarily in understanding

how one physical body moved in relation to, and was affected by, another. In the twentieth century, however, electricity became extremely important, as did eventually the study of atomic energy. More and more we came to grapple with the question, "What is the relationship between matter and energy, between the physical realm and the realm of energy phenomena?" What, in fact, is energy? If we can't see it, and it's not material, should a scientist really study it? If it can't be seen or felt, is it scientific to talk about it? Yet obviously energy is crucial. It makes us move; it makes the lights glow. Whereas our masterful machinery of a century ago burned coal to make steam and push pistons, our machinery of today has become more subtle, channeling energy through the tiniest of circuits to perform electronic miracles which have little to do with the physical, mechanical world. How can we understand this phenomen of energy?

Einstein seized this question and formulated an answer. He specified $E=mc^2$, thus stating a relationship between energy and matter. Not only does this mean that energy and matter bear a very definite relationship to each other, but it also implies that they are interconvertible. Matter can be changed into energy. The most dramatic applications of this are the atomic explosions which have snuffed out whole cities in Japan and blown entire islands off the face of the earth. Yet Einstein's formulation also implies that energy can be converted into matter. This is equally possible and equally necessary. Not only can the process move in one direction, but it can also move in the reverse direction. Energy and matter are interconvertible. Between the physical level of existence and the energy level of existence there is an intimate connection. In Sanskrit terms the level of functioning that involves energy is called, *prana*, and within the human being the Himalayan practitioners of meditation have found that there is not only a relationship between the gross physical body and the energy, or *prana*, but there is equally a relationship between *prana* and the next level higher which is the mind.

Psychologists sometimes talk about mental energy. Intuitively, and in our everyday expressions, we acknowledge the relationship between mind and energy. It is common, for instance, to experience at times a great deal of vitality and clarity of mind, while at other times one experiences a sense of having "no mental energy." Various schools of psychology have formulated this in more precise terms; Freud called this energy, for example, libido.

According to the Upanishads the various levels of existence form a continuum—the physical, the *pranic*, the mental and the higher levels of consciousness. These are layered, one upon the other. If the mind wants to affect the body, then it does it through altering the flow of energy, or *prana*. If the body affects the mind, this too is accomplished through an effect on the flow of energy which, in turn, has an impact on the mind.

Prana, then, is called the vital link between mind and body—"vital" because energy is the very basis of life and vitality. When a person dies, the energy leaves. The body is still there, but the *prana* dissipates. Here we return to the matter of breath, because breath is the vehicle for *prana*. When someone dies, and the energy and vitality have left, we say of him that he has "expired;" the breath has "gone out;" the energy has left. When someone feels more energy, more mental energy and creativity, we say of him that he has become "inspired;" there is an "inspiration." We indicate through our language an intuitive recognition of the relationship between the breath and the vital energy, its necessity for life and its necessity for creativity.

Yet this area, this level of our existence which we might call *prana*, or energy, is neglected in the Western study of man. This is an intriguing situation when we stop to think about it, for if it is true that breath influences both body and mind, then the rhythm and the rate of the breath would reflect not only one's physical condition, but it would also help to create it. It would in addition be an indication of one's emotional and mental state as well as an influence on, and a help in creating, that state. Therefore, what is going on in the totality of a person could be judged from his breathing. And this is exactly what happens. Constantly confronted with this important information, it is rather bizarre that we manage to ignore it. Here is something that takes place continually in the plain view of everyone, giving away the essence of our physical and mental states—giving away our secrets, so to speak—yet no one sees it. The most fascinating and revealing kind of information is being broadcast, but no one is receiving.

We study the mind because in the West we are preoccupied with the mental world; we are always busy with our thoughts, which we shove around like souvenirs, little bits of bric-a-brac in our heads. We almost treat them as objects which we treasure and are attached to—a reflection, no doubt, of the fact that our basic and overwhelming preoccupation is with the material world.

On the other hand, the business of energy, this matter of *prana*, we ignore completely. Yet if we were to become aware of its existence and study it, we would find that it is just as complicated as is the body, almost as complicated as the mind; it is, in fact, an extremely intricate thing. We are not talking about simply "having energy" or "not having energy." There are, rather, different qualities of energy, different patterns through which energy can flow. Qualitatively, it can vary. Quantitatively, it can vary.

In the Upanishads this *pranic* level of being is described as a "body," a second body within the physical body called the "vital body," or "vital sheath." Through it moves the vital force, or *prana*, and the Upanishads say of it, that because it dwells within the physical body, it also takes on the shape of a man. In other words, if we were able to look at each other and manage not to see the physical body at all we could, perhaps, begin to perceive that which lies within it—the energy.

At any moment in one's body, not only is matter being pushed about through veins and arteries or through the respiratory passages, and shifted around with muscular contraction and relaxation, but something else is also happening. There are changes in energy states taking place. Energy is being consumed in one place and produced or stored up in another. It is being shifted from this point to that, resulting in a net movement of energy so that we might say there is an energy "flow," and if we could stand back and look at this continually shifting picture, we would be able to map out an overall pattern of flux.

Even though we are not able to do this, we can still understand that it is there, that something of this sort must be happening.

To study this energy flow is a delicate and intricate thing, and it is for this reason that some people have spent lifetimes involved in its exploration. In the ancient literature of the yoga tradition there are entire books concerning the subject where five major *pranas* are described, each having its separate function, its way of movement. According to this, the *pranic* sheath has an extremely complex "anatomy," comprised of certain pathways, called *nadis*, through which the breath flows.

Next arises the question of how this *pranic* body is regulated and controlled so that we might discern whether there is some possibility of developing the ability to consciously and deliberately alter it. Many variables will have an impact on this pattern of energy flow. If one contracts a muscle of the arm, for instance, that has an effect on it. Energy is used up there, shifted to that part. The total overall picture changes to accommodate this. The one function which has the most central, basic and strategic impact on the energy flow, however, is that of respiration. Breathing brings in the oxygen for consumption and energy exchange. Its rate and rhythm, its course and depth of flow, all have an effect on the way the body is energized. In this way is determined whether energy will come in frequent short bursts, or in long, more gradual waves, and a pulsatory pattern of energizing is established. If we were to study this in depth we could derive a wave form that would describe both the frequency of energizing inputs as well as their amplitude.

The flow of breath, then, is constantly helping to shape the pattern of energy flow that underlies and sustains the physical body. If we can grasp what this means, if we can understand the crucial way in which the energizing effects of the breath sustain and support the metabolic processes of different parts of the body, we can begin to understand how the material, physical aspects of our gross body, its tissue functioning and the very existence of its substance, is created by, and dependent on, the process of breath. With each breath energy flows through the body in waves, and this flow of breath is constantly shaping and restructuring that pattern of energy which comprises the *pranic* body.

If we look at physiology from this point of view we begin to realize that the material body (which we have tended up to this time to regard as primary) is, in fact, secondary. Its existence is based on something more fundamental than itself. The flow of energy creates and sustains the tissues of the body, and if the energy pattern is sufficiently changed then the physical body will change. If the energy pattern is altered drastically enough the body can be completely transformed, either for better or worse.

Actually, this does happen, though ordinarily not in a very dramatic way. People do change, but they usually change in minor ways. This may be, in part, because their *characteristic* patterns of energy flow are set and self-sustaining, for breathing habits and air flow patterns (and the resulting pattern of energy flow) become very deeply grounded and established in one's life. They have a sort of momentum of their own.

However, when one sits down and deliberately

begins to work with the breathing and to manipulate it, he can gradually begin to see changes in the way his body functions, even, in some cases, in its appearance. The same thing happens when one goes through life experiences that have tremendous effects on the way the energy flows. A shock or injury, an overwhelming experience of some sort, may result in a change of posture or an alteration in the way the internal organs function. One may lose weight, for instance, his color may change, or his face and its shape become altered.

If the energy pattern shifts so that some part of the body is poorly supplied ("undernourished") with *prana*, then it will eventually become sick. It will wither and perhaps even die. A degeneration or malignancy may result. Some sort of disease process will inevitably become evident, for the tissues cannot function without the energizing that supports them. On the other hand, if one's leg is amputated some sense of still having a leg there may persist for a long while. One may even experience pain in a leg which has been amputated! He may feel that it is uncomfortable, or in the wrong position, because the energy pattern requires some time to reorganize. Some animals are able to regenerate parts that are amputated, and it would seem probable that this ability is based on the persistence of an energy flow to the area where the part was removed. The physical body is nothing more than a crystallization around the energy pattern that underlies it.

After part of a leaf, for example, is torn away the energy pattern remains—even though the physical leaf is gone. This has been demonstrated through Kirlian photography. If this pattern could be maintained long enough it is possible that the leaf would grow back and, in fact, some plants do have the capacity to regenerate in this way. Without this underlying energy field around which to structure themselves, how would cells know where to grow? The same principle is evident in the animal kingdom where we find one cell, after fertilization, growing into a complete animal, or complete person. We have tended to account for this rather simplistically by saying that cells divide and redivide until eventually the aggregate is larger and begins to differentiate. But where does this differentiation come from; how do some cells change into skin, some into muscle, while others become bone? How do they know to do that? Presumably, the information that guides the metabolism of the cell is contained in the chromosome, but each of these cells has the same chromosomal structure. Yet something is different; something guides the cells and their differentiation and their spatial arrangement. There must be a field of forces existent around which they can shape themselves.

If the level of energy, or *pranic*, function controls and gives rise to the material level of phenomena, what, we must wonder in turn, controls the energy or *pranic* level of functioning? According to the ancient writings of the Upanishads, it is said that the *pranamaya kosha*, or the energy body, is fashioned, created and regulated by a deeper or more fundamental level of existence which is called *manomaya kosha*, or mind. This mental realm of existence is even subtler than that of energy, and it is even more difficult to measure, identify and observe. But it clearly exists. Its study is the business of psychology, and as we approach it we leave the area of physiology and the subject of *prana*. Looking behind us, we discover that we have in some way bridged the mysterious gap between mind and body. Such ideas both ring true and yet are jarring to our usual way of thinking, and to understand our resulting ambivalence, it is necessary to probe a bit deeper into the difference between how the Easterner and the Westerner see themselves in relation to the universe.

Cosmic Breath:

In this scientific era of the twentieth century Western world we assume that the physical body gives rise to the mind, that the mind grows out of the body. One is born and develops a mind gradually over time. According to this view, at first in the fetus or embryo, there is no mind. Gradually, it evolves out of the physical body, and out of the physical emerge the subtler levels of existence— first energy and movement, and later, thought and consciousness. The amoeba preceded the man; the embryo precedes the conscious being. On the primordial earth molecules fell into place and life arose gradually. Over millions of years more complex forms of life arose, and eventually there emerged a conscious being like man.

But in the East, and in much of the ancient world, there has been a different way of thinking. It is exactly the opposite, in fact. It is the modern world view turned upside down, for in yoga philosophy it is said that each of the levels of being grows out of the one *above* it: Out of sheer consciousness comes the mind, a manifestation of consciousness. Out of the mind is created the necessity for a physical existence. Out of the mind and this necessity for physical existence grows a body, so in the form of a human infant this consciousness begins to manifest itself. This is a vastly different way of looking at what the world is about because it implies that the essence of our being is something beyond the physical and mental. It implies that we are all simply creations, or manifestations, of that consciousness which lies beyond the grosser levels of our existence. It is from there that we came, and it is to there that we will return. Through the process of "evolution" we drop our physical form, and even our mental being, returning to the level of purer consciousness. Out of that consciousness flows manifestation, and manifestation flows back into that consciousness. Like waves, like a tide that goes in and out, the forms take shape and disappear again. From where we stand in the physical world we might think of this as a process of expansion. All the manifestations grow out of consciousness. Then there is a process of contraction, of phenomenal manifestation whereby it's all "pulled back in."

Oddly enough, the astronomers of today are arriving at a somewhat similar view. It is the astronomer, of course, whose area of study pushes him hard up against the imponderables. His conceptualizations of the planets, galaxies, and the "geography" of the universe, force him to deal with such uncomfortable concepts as infinity and unlimited space. We can outline our solar system and stipulate our position in this galaxy. Beyond that lies the next galaxy, but after we have outlined and mapped all the galaxies of which we can see some hint, then what lies beyond that? Are there more galaxies? If so, what is beyond them? Where does it all stop, and if it does stop what is beyond that point where it stops? Suddenly we realize that our thinking is no good, that it is, in fact, childish. Somehow the astronomer has to deal with such questions. To astronomers of today, through the use of more sophisticated instrumentation, it begins to appear that the distances between galaxies are increasing, that the space between heavenly bodies is expanding. Through their calculations many of them have concluded that the galaxies and planets are pulling apart from each other, that the whole universe is swelling, so to speak. The most coherent theory at this point is that all this movement has resulted from a sort of explosion from a center. This has come to be termed the "Big Bang Theory," according to which the universe is expanding, and after a certain point it will again begin to contract and all the planets, solar systems and galaxies will be pulled back into some point from which it all explodes again.

The process, then, is a familiar one, that of expansion and contraction. It is nothing more, in a sense, than a cosmic inhalation and exhalation. The universe can be approached in these terms. All the levels of our existence can be seen as functioning harmoniously if we grasp the basic phenomenon of expansion and contraction, the "cosmic breath." On one level we manifest, we become people, we become bodies. We become physical, and then we return to consciousness. Hence it is that one can spend decades, or even a lifetime, delving into the subtleties and implications of the process of breathing.

Developing Awareness of Breath:
    The study of breath and the development of a

control over the *pranic*, or energy level of one's being, seems so shrouded in mystery. It is not actually so. In fact, the principles are very simple and scientific. The study and training in the science of breath is time-consuming only because our habits have led us away from any awareness of it, but a certain awareness of the breath can easily become a constant part of the way we function, act, feel and think.

As an analogy, one might consider the case of his left leg. Ordinarily, of course, he is not particularly worried about his left leg. At the moment he most likely is not thinking, "Oh, what shall I do with this leg next," or, "I wonder if I have put it in the proper place, this leg. Perhaps I should set it somewhere else." or "When I get up am I going to remember how to move it?" When one goes to work, he really doesn't have to stop and think, "Now the left comes after the right, the right comes next, and then the left again, and I should remember to lift the toes so they won't drag on the ground." Yet he does these things, of course. He does all that, and if he were asked at any moment, "Where's your left leg?" he would promptly reply, "Here." Of course one knows where his leg is every minute of the day, he never forgets, in fact. He never misplaces it, he always knows what it's doing. It seems, in fact, a bit amazing that one can do his work, talk and interact with the people around him and still keep up with that leg.

How is this possible? It is possible simply because for years and years we've been using our legs. At first, we should recall, it wasn't so easy. It took several years for us to learn, in fact. We started out trying to put the leg,

or at least the foot, in our mouths perhaps, playing with
it and then discovering it had feeling, that it could be
hurt, that the toes could be wiggled, and eventually finding
that we could move it, stand up on it, and even ultimately
walk on it. Soon we were walking with it every day, aware
of how to walk with it, without, as it were, giving it a
moment's thought.

It might be helpful to look at the breath in the same
way. The breath is also something of which one can be
constantly aware. A master of *pranayama*, for instance,
was once heard to remark that he was aware of every
breath he took.

The crucial point is that the breath is perhaps the
only physiological process that can be either voluntary or
involuntary. One can breathe, making his breath do whatever he wishes, or he can ignore it, and after a while the
body simply begins to breathe on its own. Breathing
becomes reflexive. The body can't operate without breath,
so if conscious control of the breath is abandoned, then
some unconscious part of the mind begins functioning,
picks it up and starts breathing for us. Something is
triggered in the lower part of the brain that stimulates the
breathing. So if the breath is ignored, breathing will go on
anyhow. But in this case breathing falls back to control
by primitive parts of the brain, the unconscious realms
of the mind where emotions, thoughts and feelings (of
which we may have little or no awareness) become involved, and they wreak havoc with the rhythms of the
breath. In other words, the breath becomes haphazard and
often irregular if we lose conscious control of it.

The same thing, of course, can happen with one's

left leg. There are people who pay no attention to their legs; they simply walk on them and are never very aware of them. Often, as a result, they develop problems with their feet because of the way they are used (or rather, misused). The foot is neglected, lost from attention, there is no awareness of it, no consciousness of it. Instead of feeling and registering, "Oh, there's too much pressure on that side," and making an adjustment, one simply goes ahead and walks on it. Then he develops various foot problems, and the foot becomes twisted and distorted. If you take such a person, train him to do foot exercises and slowly bring the foot back into his awareness, it may begin to function properly and heal.

The same thing happens with the breath. It can either be allowed to run haphazardly and create havoc in the body and the mind which it influences, or, on the other hand, it can become a part of one's constant awareness and be harmoniously coordinated. And once the breath becomes a part of one's awareness, he begins to wonder how he ever managed to live when he was ignoring it.

Something similar will sometimes happen with a person who has had an injury and cannot walk for some time. Often he will develop the habit of simply ignoring the lower half of the body. He lives from the waist up. What's above the waist is alive and that below is just a weight which is dragged about. Now if it happens that he recovers functioning of the lower half of the body, then he must go through an elaborate process of learning how to walk and how to use the legs again. It becomes a completely new matter to get the lower half of the body back into one's awareness—to extend oneself back down into the legs, and this requires work because one has developed the mental habit of "throwing that part of himself away," ignoring it, cutting it off. As far as his awareness goes, it has ceased to exist.

And here is the problem that we begin to confront when we learn about breathing. We must bring back into our awareness a whole area of ourselves that we've cut off. We have acted as though it didn't exist, as though it's not part of us, so gradually it must be re-integrated into our consciousness. The more we make it part of our constant awareness, the more it becomes a dimension of ourselves.

At that point we begin to understand the teachings about *pranayama*, the recommendations that are made about when one should inhale through one nostril, when he should exhale through the other, and so forth. Through constant awareness and experience we discover for ourselves what happens when we breathe through one nostril or the other. When the breath flows through one nostril there is a certain total feeling, both in the mind and in the body. When the breath shifts there is a shift of feeling *tone*. Having lunch today with the left nostril open, for instance, is followed by the realization that the food doesn't sit quite as well as usual. A constant awareness of the breath provides such experiences. "My stomach feels a bit uneasy and I think I know why," one realizes. It is said in the scriptures that one should eat only when the right nostril is open. If the emotions are so closely related to the breath, then altering the rhythms of the breath should shift emotional gears. This need not remain a hypothesis. It is something we can try out, experiment

with, from moment to moment. In this way the science of
breath ceases to be mere theory. It's no longer merely a
matter of something read in a book. It becomes part of
one's total awareness and experience, another dimension
of his existence.

But this awareness of breath, as an added dimension
of one's experience, comes only gradually. The stage for
this is set by an understanding of the breath and by the
regular practice of breath awareness and breathing
exercises. The result is an awakening of a whole part of
oneself that he didn't know was there before; a completely
new aspect of his being, his life and his living to which his
eyes before had been closed.

Two

Respiration and the Chest

Alan Hymes, M.D.

In day-to-day life few basic physiological functions have escaped the attention of modern man to the degree that breathing has. The importance of the heart, for instance, is known to everyone, largely because of the prevalence of coronary artery disease. Similarly, one can observe present-day concerns with the digestive organs by noting the bewildering array of commercial preparations centered upon modifying their activity. In contrast, except for diseases associated with smoking, the organs of breathing have been largely ignored. Considering that one can readily modify the flow of breath, whereas the control and functioning of other internal organs remains inaccessible to the average person, this is all the more surprising.

Knowledge of the dynamics of breathing, however, need not be shrouded in ignorance. By understanding a few basic principles of how the breathing process operates and interacts with the body and mind, one can readily gain some clear and intensely practical insight into previously unknown levels of functioning, for the movement of muscles to transport air in and out of the body is only the grossest manifestation of the breathing process. The effects of breathing extend to the workings of the heart and lungs as well as to subtle physiological interactions such as the molecular processes through which the body's energy production is maintained.

Cellular Respiration:

All organisms, human or plant or animal, are composed of a multitude of tiny individual living units called cells, and it is these cells and the manner in which they are organized into specific tissues and organs, that form the physical body. This organization—the very life of these individual cells and therefore the body as a whole—is dependent upon a continuous source of energy.

We usually think of the food we eat as supplying our energy needs in terms of a certain amount of carbohydrate, protein and fat, but these nutrients are actually useless to the body as sources of energy unless they can be converted into a form which can be used by its cells. In other words, it is often said that we burn carbohydrate in the body, but what does this mean? If carbohydrate is being burned in my tissues, why doesn't it hurt? Why doesn't my fat sizzle? Where does the smoke go, and the ash for that matter? If I exercise vigorously in a dark room, shouldn't I be able to see my body glow from the light produced by the burning carbohydrate? It is said that the body is 88% water. How can I burn carbohydrate under water when I can't even get a campfire started when the wood is damp?

In a fire, energy is released in the form of heat and light. The reaction involves the burning of carbon-containing substances, and if this burning is efficient the end result is the formulation of carbon dioxide gas (CO_2), water and ash, along with the release of energy. The energy which is produced when something burns quickly is usually manifested as heat and light.

The heat energy in a fire, or explosion, can be used to drive a machine such as a steam engine, but an automobile engine is driven by a more rapid burning process—gasoline exploding in a chamber. Here, one wall of the chamber, or cylinder, is pushed by the explosion, and thus a coordinated series of controlled explosions in multiple chambers turns a shaft which in turn moves the wheels of the car.

How then do our bodies harness energy? Cells must have energy, but they do not run on explosions. All living organisms can be thought of as meeting their energy needs from a slow-burning furnace. This furnace releases energy from a constant supply of fuel by slowly combining it with oxygen. In a rapidly burning system oxygen (O_2) present in the air combines instantly with fuel so that a readily visible fire results. The products of this burning are CO_2, water, heat and light, and in very rapidly burning systems this reaction can be quite dramatic, as in a firecracker exploding. However, when fuel is consumed more slowly, energy is also produced but at a slower rate, yielding a steady flame. If the rate is very slow, there may be no light visible at all. Biological systems (i.e., all living organisms) are essentially burning fuel at a very slow rate.

The fuel that we use comes from the carbohydrates and fats that we eat, and the energy released by combination with oxygen must take place under very special circumstances to keep it in a form that is both useful and safe. That is why the reaction takes place in tiny subunits within the cell, called mitochondrias. These contain a series of specialized protein molecules, or enzymes, called the cytochrome oxidase system which takes the energy released from the oxidation of our food and transfers it to an energy storage molecule called adenosine triphosphate, or ATP. Found in biological systems throughout nature, for practical purposes ATP may be thought of as the basic unit of energy storage for cells. It has the ability to deliver energy within the cells of the body which, in turn, maintains the chemical reactions necessary for the cells to function normally.

The actual process of respiration, then, occurs within the cell where nutrient fuel is burned with oxygen to release energy. The nose, trachea (windpipe), lungs, circulatory system and their attendant muscles all act to transport or modify O_2 from the surrounding air to make it readily available to individual cells within the body. Each of these organs plays a crucial role in determining oxygen supply, and therefore energy availability, to cells at various levels within the body. A change in functioning in any one of these systems could therefore potentially alter the course of energy production within the body.

Pulmonary and Circulatory Systems:

In order for oxygen to be available in the cell for respiration, it undergoes an interesting journey from the atmosphere through the lungs and circulatory system and finally into the cell.

As air is inhaled through the nose and into the chest it encounters the main airway leading to the lungs, the trachea. This is a smooth, tubelike structure beginning just below the larynx, or "Adam's apple." Shortly thereafter it splits into two smaller tubes, one supplying each lung. These airways, called bronchi, branch off like limbs on a tree, getting smaller and smaller until they become microscopic in size. After about fifteen "generations," or branching levels, they terminate in tiny brochioles, and each of these, in turn, ends in a series of tiny little air sacs called alveoli. These air sacs are so tiny that lung tissue actually looks solid and fleshy to the naked eye. In reality, however, the alveoli are much like bubbles. They have very thin walls—only one cell thick—and these cells, too, are very thin and membranous. It is here that the gas exchange occurs.

Surrounding the alveoli is a network of tiny blood vessels—capillaries so thin that blood cells literally have to squeeze through them, bending to fit through. By breathing, O_2 in the air moves down the trachea, through the bronchial system, into alveoli where it flows into the blood stream that is within the capillaries surrounding the alveoli.

For this process to take place efficiently there should ideally be a balance between the amount of blood flowing within the capillaries to absorb oxygen and the amount of oxygen brought to the alveolus by breathing. The casual observer might say, "Well, that's obvious." But the physiology of the lung shows that blood is not evenly distributed throughout the entire lung field. It is gravity-dependent, and in the upright position there is far more blood in the lower part of the lung than in the upper part. However, the free flow of gases into and out

The Bronchial Tree

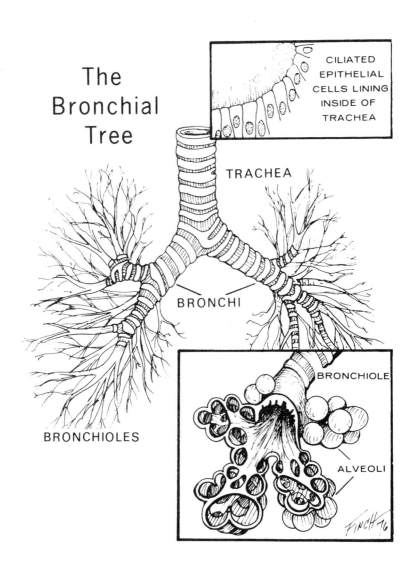

CILIATED EPITHELIAL CELLS LINING INSIDE OF TRACHEA

TRACHEA

BRONCHI

BRONCHIOLE

ALVEOLI

BRONCHIOLES

FINCH 76

of the alveoli is greater in the upper portions of the lung, so this process of oxygen transfer (from the air into the blood) is not necessarily as efficient as it appears at first glance. The degree of inefficiency can be reduced not only by compensating reflexes in the lungs, but also by the way in which we habitually breathe.

More serious inefficiencies develop if the alveoli become injured, as they do from smoking, for if the lining of the many tiny alveoli is broken down, what was once an area consisting of multiple small chambers becomes one larger pocket which appears as a visible hole in the lung tissue. If this happens, the tremendous surface area in which oxygen comes into contact with blood is significantly reduced and results in a condition called emphysema. It develops slowly and silently, over a period of years because of noxious fumes being taken into the lungs, breaking down the delicate walls of the alveoli. The most common cause of emphysema is cigarette smoking, and it is such a problem that several million Americans are crippled by it. All smokers have emphysema to some degree, but because of the enormous area that exists for diffusion of O_2 most people are not aware that they have this condition during their everyday activities. Most people have about three hundred million alveoli in their lungs (and if one could flatten each of these out and lay them side by side they would cover an area greater than an average one-bedroom apartment). It is only when this area becomes drastically reduced that one finds he cannot exchange enough gas to keep up with his oxygen needs when they increase. He will notice this during exercise, for example, and feel "short of breath."

Oxygen, once it gets into the bloodstream, into the busy capillaries, can be transported by two basic mechanisms: it can either be bound by the hemoglobin molecule within red blood cells or it can be directly dissolved in the blood, but practically all of the oxygen which is transported through the bloodstream is carried by hemoglobin. This molecule is composed of four protein chains attached to one atom of iron, and it is this iron atom to which O_2 gas is attracted and which facilitates their transport throughout the circulation (when O_2 is bound to this iron atom it turns the freshly oxygenated blood a fiery red). Hemoglobin can also carry CO_2, a "waste" product from cells, which it picks up for the return trip to the heart and lungs after it has delivered its O_2. The combination of CO_2 with hemoglobin, along with the loss of oxygen, gives a bluish color to the blood, and this, of course, is why arterial blood is bright red and venous blood bluish.

Normally O_2 and CO_2 should be the only molecules which bind to hemoglobin. However, some other gases present in the environment can enter the bloodstream via the lungs and also be bound, essentially crowding out the O_2 from the hemoglobin. A very common substance that does exactly this is carbon monoxide, which appears in high concentrations in both cigarette smoke and automobile exhaust fumes. Having an affinity for hemoglobin that is 240 times that of O_2, carbon monoxide latches on to a hemoglobin molecule, and since the carbon monoxide removes the hemoglobin from the O_2 transport system, this results in a decreased amount of hemoglobin available to carry O_2 —or a relative "anemia." So one who smokes cigarettes may have from five to fifteen percent of all his hemoglobin tied up with carbon monoxide at any given time, even if he is not smoking at that time.

The problem actually goes further than that because carbon monoxide may also contribute to hardening of the arteries, or arteriosclerotic disease. The exact mechanism by which carbon monoxide gives rise to this disease process is not completely understood although it has been observed both clinically and experimentally, but the death rate in smokers from heart attacks and strokes is approximately three to five times greater than the death rate in non-smokers.

Once hemoglobin molecules are oxygenated, they still have to travel throughout the body in order to supply the needs of individual cells, and the driving force which propels blood throughout the body is, of course, the heart. This is divided into two separate functional sections: The right side takes oxygen-poor (CO_2 rich) venous blood from the body and pumps it into the capillaries surrounding the lung's alveoli where gas exchange occurs. Then this newly oxygenated arterial blood is redistributed throughout the body by the left side of the heart. As the oxygenated blood approaches the cells along its route of travel, it moves through increasingly smaller vessels to the point at which red blood cells squeeze through capillaries that are the same size as those found surrounding the alveoli in the lungs. This time, however, the capillaries surround cells in other parts of the body (muscles, nerves, etc.), and at this point gas exchange similar to that which takes place in the lungs occurs—but now it is between the hemoglobin and a cell. Here, waste CO_2 from the cell is exchanged for O_2 from the red blood cell hemoglobin, depleting the blood of O_2 and thereby turning it blue. This newly made venous blood then travels through a series of successively increasingly larger veins, eventually going through the right side of the heart and winding up back in the lungs to complete the cycle again.

The Mechanics of Breathing:

Previously, the respiratory system has been discussed in terms of levels which are not readily visible to the casual observer: molecular interactions, microscopic transport and internal anatomy. The focus of discussion now shifts closer to the body's surface in order to study the organization and action of those structures which create the driving force for moving air in and out of the body.

In looking at the body, several anatomical divisions become readily apparent—the four limbs, the head and the torso. Each comprise distinct anatomical units. Since it is the torso which contains the organs responsible for movement of air into the body, as well as the other major organ systems responsible for distribution of O_2, it is here that a discussion of the mechanics of breathing must be centered.

One can subdivide the torso into three regions: the thorax, or chest, which houses the heart and two lungs; the abdomen, which begins immediately below the thorax and is separated from it by a sheet of muscle, the diaphragm, and contains the organs of digestion; and, finally, the pelvis, which extends from the hip bones down to the bottom of the torso, housing the organs of excretion and reproduction. The pelvis will, for the purposes of this discussion, be considered as essentially continuous with the abdomen.

Looking only at the supporting bone, muscle and skin, with the internal organs removed, the torso can be viewed as forming a rough cylinder, slightly flattened out, so that it is wider than it is deep when seen in cross section. The bony spine, or vertebral column, which runs vertically through the back parallel to the long axis of the torso "cylinder," provides structural support for the whole torso, acting as a framework around which other tissues and organs are grouped. The vertebral column itself is composed of a number of small individual bones called vertebrae. They are stacked, one on top of the other, and are separated by discs of shock absorbing tissue. The first twelve of these bones within the torso, the thoracic vertebrae, each attach to a pair of ribs, one on either side. The ribs all travel parallel to each other, curving in a forward and downward direction, and the first ten join in the midline and fuse with the sternum, or breastbone, to form a "cage of ribs." Connecting the ribs and vertebrae together is a series of small joints which allows them to move slightly in a hinged fashion, somewhat like a curved bucket handle moves. The ribs, along with their attachments to the sternum in front and vertebral column in back, form the walls of the thoracic, or chest, portion of the body cylinder.

Since the ribs, in actuality, gradually increase in length of curvature from top to bottom of the thorax, the widest part of the thorax occurs at its lower margin, and attached to these lower ribs and to the sternum and vertebral column is a tough flat sheet of muscle—the diaphragm. In effect, it divides the torso cylinder into two smaller cylinders, one stacked on top of the other—the chest cavity above and the abdominal cavity below. The boundaries of the abdominal cylinder include the vertebral column and its supporting muscles in the back and the floor of the pelvis, both of which are relatively inflexible and fixed, and the abdominal contents, lying just beneath the surface of the diaphragm, extend partly into the chest cavity. Several overlapping sheets of muscle, extending from the ribs above to the pelvis below, form the front and sides of the abdomen.

The diaphragm, which separates the chest and abdominal cavities, is not flat in its resting position, but rather it billows up into the chest cavity somewhat like a parachute, or dome. For this reason its movements are not directly visible at the body's surface, and one has to infer its activity based upon the effects its movements have on other body tissues.

Immediately above the diaphragm are the right and left lungs, and nestled between them, the heart. The lungs do not actually touch the diaphragm directly, for they are completely covered with a very thin double layer of tissue known as pleura. Normally, these two layers are in direct contact with each other, slightly moistened by a small amount of pleural fluid which acts as a lubricant, allowing the pleural layers to freely slide over each other.

The innermost pleural layer completely covers the outside of each lung, while the outer layer covers the inner surface of the chest wall and the thoracic side of the diaphragm. Since both pleural layers are in such close contact with one another, a movement of the chest wall, or diaphragm, will be transmitted to the lungs, and vice versa. If, for instance, the diaphragm moves downward or the ribs expand outward, the lungs will follow, expanding in the process. These are, in fact, the two main mechanisms by which air moves into the lungs.

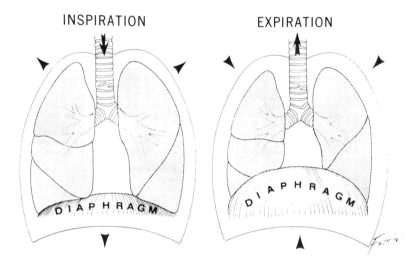

Air flow into the lungs occurs when the structures surrounding them expand and pull the lungs along with them. The resulting suction pulls air into the lungs from the upper airways to the trachea and bronchial tree into the alveoli, and the process of inhalation occurs.

Thinking of the chest cavity as a cylinder again, one can produce an increase in its volume, and consequently inhalation, by one of three means: extending the diaphragmatic floor of the cylinder downward, expanding the walls outward, or moving the top of the cylinder upward. These three phases of breathing will be termed: diaphragmatic; thoracic, or chest; and clavicular breathing. As will be seen, these three phases occur in sequence when one breathes to maximum capacity as in the complete yogic breath.

Diaphragmatic inhalation, then, is accomplished by moving the diaphragm downward. How is this done? Why does it move down? The diaphragm, as all muscles, can assume two states, an active contracted state when the individual muscle fibers shorten, or a passive relaxed state in which muscle fibers achieve a maximum length. In its relaxed state the diaphragm is shaped like a domed parachute with its rounded surface bulging upward. During contraction the remaining "slack" is taken up when the individual muscle fibers contract. The diaphragm then tends to assume the smallest surface area possible, which, since it is attached to the edges of the thoracic cylinder, flattens it from a dome to a disc. This markedly increases chest cavity's volume. But as the diaphragm moves down it decreases the volume of the abdominal cavity, so if the abdominal wall is relaxed, it moves passively outward, reestablishing the volume needed for the abdominal organs.

Of the three types of breathing mentioned, diaphragmatic breathing is physiologically the most efficient. A major portion of the blood circulating in the lungs goes to the lower portions, or gravity-dependent parts, and expansion occurs in these lower portions (although all of the lung expands to some degree). Since one of the

Synergistic Effect of Rectus Abdominus Muscle and Diaphragm on Forced Expiration

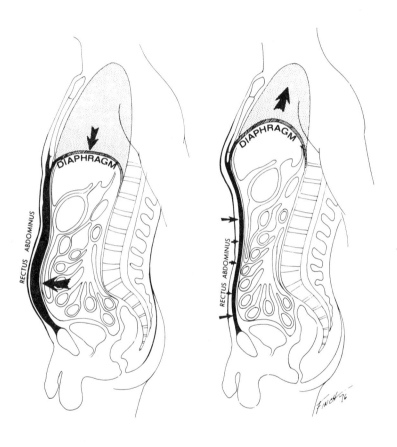

Inspiration   Expiration

purposes of breathing is to expose the blood in the capillaries to air, diaphragmatic breathing in the upright
position is very efficient. It is also interesting to note that
infants and small children use their diaphragms exclusively
for breathing. Chest breathing cannot occur until considerably after birth, not until after the bony chest matures.

A second major way of moving air into the lungs is to
expand the diameter of the thorax which involves moving
the ribs around their joints of attachment to the vertebrae.
A specialized group of muscles, the intercostals (Latin for
between the ribs), performs this function, and many
people have experienced these muscles as the "meat"
sandwiched between the bones of barbequed ribs. These
muscles exist in two layers, external and internal. The
external are aligned in such a way as to actually swing the
ribs upward and forward, pivoting them around their joints
with the vertebrae. This increases the diameter of the chest,
and the lungs consequently expand, pulling air into the
alveoli to fill the newly-created space. The internal intercostals perform exactly the opposite function, pulling the
ribs down and in, effecting a reduction in lung volume.

Chest breathing fills the middle and upper portion
of the lungs with air but is not so efficient with the lower
portion. When the body is upright, however, most of the
blood is in the lower, gravity-dependent areas and so
air is not mixed as thoroughly with blood if breathing is
done by expanding the ribs. Chest breathing also requires
more work to accomplish the same blood/gas mixing
than does slow, deep diaphragmatic breathing, and since
more work is required, more O_2 is needed, resulting in
one's taking more frequent breaths. Finally, more blood

needs to circulate through the lungs, requiring more work from the heart. How much work the cardiovascular system must do, then, is directly related to how efficiently one breathes.

The third type of inhalation, clavicular, is only significant when the maximum amount of air is needed. Its name derives from the two clavicles, or collarbones, which are pulled up slightly at the end of maximum inhalation, for this movement expands and lengthens the very top of the thoracic cylinder, and thus the very top of the lungs. Clavicular breathing only comes into play when the body's oxygen demands are very great.

The three types of inhalation can be coordinated into one smooth exercise in which a maximum deep breath is taken. This is the yogic complete breath which has a diaphragmatic, thoracic and clavicular phase. It is initiated by diaphragmatic contraction, resulting in a slight expansion of the lower ribs and protrusion of the upper abdomen, thus oxygenating the lower lung fields. Then the middle portions of the lungs expand, with outward chest movement, in the thoracic phase as inhalation proceeds further. At the very end of inhalation still more air is admitted by slightly raising the clavicles, thereby expanding the uppermost tips of the lungs. In sequence, then, each phase of inhalation acts on one particular area of the lungs.

Now that the lungs are filled to their capacity with air, how are they emptied? What results in exhalation? Relaxation! Everyone has had the experience of sighing, or letting a deep breath out in a completely relaxed, passive motion. No muscles contracted to push the air out. It was as if the lungs themselves were pulling the diaphragm and chest wall in. This is in fact, what happens. The lungs act as if they were elastic, and they shrink back to their original size once the forces which expanded them are released—much as a balloon shrinks back to its normal size once the end is untied.

The reason for this elastic recoil is quite fascinating. Again like a balloon, the lung has some elastic fibers in its tissue. But more important, the elasticity is related to the millions upon millions of tiny rounded pockets of cells, the alveoli. Each one of these alveoli is coated inside by a thin layer of protein-containing fluid called surfactant, which is the secret behind the lung's elastic properties, for surfactant possesses a property, common to all fluids, known as surface tension. This can be illustrated by looking at a soap bubble. The walls of the bubble, being mostly water with some dissolved soap, are liquid. As one blows on the bubble the trailing edges snap together to form a sphere while the surface layer of the soapy water exerts a force, or tension, drawing it together to assume the smallest area possible—which in three dimensions is a bubble. Surface tension then continues to maintain this round shape. For the same reason, beads of water and other liquids tend to assume a rounded shape.

In the lungs, the effects of surface tension are very important, considering the large area covered by surfactant, for in order for inhalation to occur the muscles involved must overcome the effects of surface tension in order to expand the lungs. Once the muscles relax, however, surface tension is unopposed; the lungs are drawn together, and the chest and diaphragm follow suit. The intercostal and abdominal muscles can, of course, augment exhalation, speeding up, or deepening, the process, but it is the lung's ability to recoil on its own that is of crucial importance. People whose respiratory muscles, with the exception of the diaphragm, are all paralyzed, can still inhale and exhale without assistance, for surface tension provides sufficient opposition to the diaphragm to maintain breathing by itself.

This explains why the relaxed diaphragm billows upward like a parachute instead of sagging into the abdomen, pulled down by gravity; surface tension within the lungs keeps them contracted when the respiratory muscles are relaxed. This force is stronger than gravity, and the diaphragm thus remains supported, pulled upward by the lungs via the pleural layers. There are interesting differences in the interplay between diaphragmatic motion and gravity, depending upon the posture one assumes. If the body is in an upright posture, gravity tends to pull downward on the abdominal contents, the diaphragm and the lungs, opposing the elastic recoil of the lungs and facilitating the downward movement of the diaphragm during inhalation.

When one lies flat on his back the diaphragm is oriented vertically, with respect to the floor, and pushes the abdominal wall upward when it contracts during inhalation, requiring a slightly increased force of diaphragmatic contraction. During exhalation gravity can then act to pull this abdominal bulge downward when the diaphragm relaxes, and the abdominal contents, no longer pushed by the diaphragm against gravity, move against the flaccid diaphragm, helping to restore it to its original resting position. Little or no muscular effort is needed to counterbalance diaphragmatic inhalation contraction in this position.

Complete exhalation beyond the position at which the diaphragm is at rest requires active muscular effort in opposition to that involved in a complete breath—except that the diaphragm no longer takes part. Since a muscle can only contract in one direction, a second muscle, or force, is required for active movement in the opposite direction. Looking at the three phases of breathing that take place in the complete breath, three opposing sets of forces are necessary for extreme exhalation. Therefore several muscles are attached to the clavicles, and one can clearly define muscle groups which act to either elevate or depress them for a full cycle of inhalation/exhalation. Similarly, the external intercostals are paired with the internal intercostals, each group opposing the action of the other in the thoracic phase of breathing.

There is, however, no muscle or group of muscles which are paired with the diaphragm to produce muscular contraction in exactly the opposite direction, but a set of muscles does exist which can act to achieve a similar effect. These are the abdominal muscles—four layers of muscle which crisscross over each other to form the front and side walls of the abdomen. Just as the diaphragm pushes the abdominal organs downward, causing the abdomen to bulge forward during diaphragmatic contraction, so do the abdominal muscles contracting cause the opposite effect to take place. Contraction of the abdominal wall pushes the abdominal organs upward against a relaxed diaphragm during exhalation, causing it to rise upward beyond its resting position, compressing and emptying the lung more completely than could the diaphragm alone.

Breathing Habits:

We have seen that the breathing process has an influence upon various levels of the organism, from subtle molecular interactions in the energization of ATP by O_2, to the grosser physical movements which propel air in and out of the lungs. Of these levels the most visible, and the one with which we identify most closely, is the physical motion of the chest and abdomen. To breathe is before all else to move air into and out of the body, and the motion of chest and diaphragm is the essential first step in determining the amount and manner in which O_2 is delivered for respiration.

That the quantity of air taken into the body is important is obvious. Not enough air and consequently insufficient O_2 to meet the body's energy demands will result in a reduction, or even cessation, of cellular functioning, ending in death. Less obvious, but of great importance in maintaining health, is the quality of the breathing process—that is, the manner in which air is inspired and expired. Whether breathing is diaphragmatic or thoracic, continuous or interrupted by pauses, rhythmical or irregular, can be of major significance in determining one's physical and emotional state,* and by looking at a single specific breathing characteristic, or group of

---

* For more details on this subject see Swami Rama, Rudolph Ballentine, M. D., and Swami Ajaya, *Yoga and Psychotherapy* (Honesdale, PA: the Himalayan Institute), 1976, pp. 34-37.

characteristics, one can then speak of different breathing modes, or habits. Everyone has had some experience with a disruption in breathing pattern associated with pain or powerful emotions. A sob of grief, a startled gasp, and the deep trembling breaths of one in anger are well known examples of how emotion can affect breathing. But the relationship extends beyond this, for a change in the breathing pattern can also alter an emotional state as well as effect physiological changes in the body. An examination of some common breathing habits will clarify this.

During average daily activities, most people employ a variant of either chest or diaphragmatic breathing, predominantly. The maximum inhalation of the complete breath can be performed for short periods of time as a breathing exercise, or during heavy physical activity when O_2 requirements are high, but it is otherwise rarely encountered.

Of the various types of breathing, the one best suited for everyday relaxed functioning is diaphragmatic breathing. Here, lung expansion is focused on the lower gravity-dependent areas of the lung where oxygen exchange can proceed more efficiently. The diaphragm performs its function well, not only in adults, but also in infants and young children where it is the sole muscle of inhalation. In addition to providing the most efficient breathing pattern, the diaphragm, as it contracts, pushes the abdominal organs down and forward, and this rhythmical massage gently compresses the abdominal organs, promoting improved circulation.

In addition to being an excellent regular mode of

functioning, diaphragmatic breathing has shown potential as a therapeutic tool in dealing with several abnormalities. Essential hypertension (high blood pressure of unknown cause) has been shown to respond favorably to a daily regimen of diaphragmatic breathing.* This is especially encouraging when one considers the number of deaths per year in the U.S. from heart disease alone, that are associated with hypertension. Diaphragmatic breathing, in conjunction with relaxation exercises, has resulted in impressive improvements in treating anxiety states in at least one study, and this represents a mode of treatment free from the potential side effects of medications. The application of such a simple, safe and inexpensive method as an adjunct to other therapies is an exciting one for further research.

A second type of breathing, chest breathing, occurs very frequently in our society. Here chest wall movement, rather than diaphragmatic movement, is the major component of breathing. Expansion is therefore centered at the mid-portion of the lungs, and gas exchange is consequently less efficient than in diaphragmatic breathing. For a number of reasons, too, there is evidence to indicate that anxiety is more frequently associated with chest breathing as opposed to diaphragmatic breathing if it is employed as the major resting breathing pattern. A number of therapists, notably from Alexander Lowens' school of bioenergetics place great importance on breathing,† maintaining that many people actually "freeze," or

---

*For further details see James Funderburk, Ph.D., *Science Studies Yoga* (Honesdale, PA: Himalayan Institute), 1977, pp. 36-41.
† See *Yoga and Psychotherapy*, pp. 246-248.

immobilize, their diaphragms instead, using their bodies to breathe in an attempt to contain fears of aggression and other powerful feelings and keep them out of consciousness. Since psychoanalysts hold that emotions centered on sex, fear and aggression have strong associations with lower parts of the body, stiffening the diaphragm can serve to isolate the associated feelings in the lower body, pushing them out of awareness.

It has also been suggested that chest breathing relates to our popular conceptions of body image. Normal diaphragmatic breathing pushes the abdomen forward during inhalation, but unfortunately a protruding abdomen is not fashionable in our society. The wide shoulders of an athlete, tapering to a thin waist, and the hour-glass figure of a bathing beauty represent the epitome of popular beauty, so many people push out their chest and pull in the abdomen, keeping it tense, thereby limiting diaphragmatic movement. This could lead to an increased reliance upon chest breathing to supply the body's O_2 requirements as well as producing chronic muscle tension in the chest and abdomen.

A physiological theory has also been proposed in an attempt to relate anxiety and chest breathing. Whenever physical or emotional stress, such as a sports event, an emotional crisis or an unavoidable accident is anticipated, the body gears up its defense mechanisms and prepares to deal with the confrontation by either "flight or fight." The response is one we have all experienced at some time and is characterized by cold sweaty palms, a pounding heart and acute anxiety. Coordination of this response is achieved by the autonomic nervous system—that network which controls the functioning of those internal organs and tissues which do not require constant conscious input in order to operate smoothly (e.g. heart, liver, kidneys, bowels, etc.). Anatomically and physiologically, the autonomic nervous system is divided into two branches, the parasympathetic and sympathetic systems. The former is involved in controlling resting activities: slowing the heart rate, speeding up digestion and activating the cleansing processes of the body. In contrast, the sympathetic system regulates more active, externally directed functions such as those involved in responding to emergency situations or physical exercise.* When the sympathetic nervous system is activated, the heart rate increases and blood is shunted away from the digestive and excretory organs to the muscles of the limbs, readying the body for physical activity. The balance between sympathetic and parasympathetic systems is reciprocal and determines the overall state of the autonomic nervous system at a given moment.

Breathing, also under autonomic control, becomes accentuated during the "fight or flight" response, and even where diaphragmatic breathing may have predominated earlier, chest breathing now also appears to meet the anticipated increased oxygen needs. If the anticipated event results in physical activity, the body is prepared and discharges its accumulated energy, but if not, hyperventilation, in association with anxiety, is commonly

---

* For further details on sympathetic arousal see Swami Ajaya, ed., *Meditational Therapy* (Honesdale, PA: The Himalayan Institute), 1977, p. 37 ff.

seen. In this case an increased amount of air is exchanged by the blood stream due to excessive breathing. If no physical activity has occurred to achieve a balance in gas exchange, and if the "red warning lights" continue to flash in one's head, the physical symptoms, anxiety state and excessive breathing continue. In susceptible people this hyperventilation alone can cause a metabolic derangement resulting in irritability and/or lightheadedness, and a further increase in anxiety.

It has been suggested that by chronic chest breathing one can perpetuate or recreate a state of sympathetic nervous system "arousal," recreating the above situation. For this reason, studying the interrelationship between emotions, breath and the autonomic nervous system could potentially yield valuable insights into the prevention and treatment of numerous diseases.

Still another major breathing type, paradoxical breathing, involves a combination of expanding the chest while simultaneously contracting the abdominal muscles which pushes the diaphragm up into the chest cavity. Although the chest wall expands, increasing lung volume, the diaphragm simultaneously rises and diminishes these gains. It is immediately obvious that this cannot be an efficient way to breathe, fighting against oneself for air. Then why would anyone breathe this way?

Although breathing is partly under voluntary control, as mentioned earlier, it is also regulated by the autonomic nervous system, and any attempt to breathe consciously in a manner which threatens survival (for instance, holding the breath beyond one's capacity) is overridden by this regulatory system. Responses to many emotions are also involuntary. The symptoms of acute anxiety, the "blush" of embarrassment and a trembling fit of rage are expressed directly by the autonomic nervous system, often bypassing conscious control. We can all identify how we characteristically respond to specific emotions time after time. That we have these reactions in common with the experiences of most other people indicates a common fundamental psychophysiological response.

Paradoxical breathing is seen in conjunction with a sudden shock or surprise. One reflexively gasps when startled, expanding the chest while tensing the abdomen. If a situation which elicits paradoxical breathing occurs frequently, either because of the presence of much stimulation from the environment or because of an excessive sensitivity to environmental cues, the body will accommodate to this mode of functioning, gradually offering less and less resistance to it. Then, after being accustomed to this abnormal pattern, the very real danger exists of the body becoming less specific in its application of this pattern. Relatively minor stresses may then also begin to initiate the same response. And if, as has been previously suggested, breathing itself is intimately associated with and can, in turn, reinforce or recreate the original emotional atmosphere, a vicious cycle ensues. Either the emotion or breath occurs in association with the other. Breathing therapy then becomes much more complicated than simply dealing with a set of muscular movements. It becomes a potential tool for intervention in interrupting or controlling undesired emotional response patterns.

Another way to look at breathing is to observe

the quality of breath flow. Is it smooth and continuous or is it irregular and choppy? Based upon one's own experiences, one can see that emotions can profoundly affect this flow. Sorrow, pain, anger, for instance, each disrupt the smooth, relaxed pattern. As with other types of breathing, irregularities in flow also tell something of the state of the physical body. This is especially true of apneic disturbances, or "interruptions," in the flow of breath. These breathing pauses can occur at various points in the cycle of inhalation/exhalation, varying in duration from a fraction of a second to a minute, and occurring during both sleep and wakefulness.

Of the different possible types of breathing pauses, sleep apnea has recently received much attention in popular and medical circles. In this syndrome breathing pauses, lasting up to one minute in severe cases, occur throughout the sleep. As one would expect, this has definite detrimental effects on health, at least in its extreme forms, for the breathing pauses are often accompanied by elevated blood pressure and a decrease in blood O_2 levels. The latter may fall to such low levels, in fact, that one actually turns blue for a few seconds, and in over half of one group of patients studied, the blood pressure remained elevated throughout the day. Various psychological traits were also noted in people with sleep apnea. Anxiety, occasional confusion, depression and decreased sexual drive as well as diminished mentation occurred more frequently in those who had extreme cases of sleep apnea.

This is a fascinating bit of information, but it was thought not to be of much practical value, considering the small number of people with sleep apnea. However, recently a study examining "normal" hospital staff volunteers found that two thirds of the men had periods of sleep apnea, in association with low blood O_2 levels, lasting longer than ten seconds. Oddly enough, only a very small number of women experienced any apneic periods at all, none of these associated with low O_2 levels.

The high incidence of sleep apnea in men and the disparity between the sexes in this regard has yet to be systematically explored, though some tentative theories exist. For instance, the association of sleep apnea with periods of low blood oxygenation levels and elevated blood pressure suggests that heart functioning may be affected. The heart is composed of several muscular chambers whose function is to propel blood throughout the body. If the blood pressure is elevated the heart must work harder, using more O_2 to pump the same amount of blood against this increased resistance. If, at the same time, blood O_2 levels fall, as in sleep apnea, this could create a temporary energy shortage for the heart. Repeating this process frequently, every night for years, could conceivably have a cumulative adverse effect on heart functioning. If one then considers that the death rate from heart disease is much higher in men than in women, might the incidence of heart disease and sleep apnea be related? Does sleep apnea causally affect the development of heart disease? Can modification of this breathing type then exert a therapeutic or preventative effect on the development of heart disease?

These questions have yet to be answered. There is, however, some evidence to support the need for further research into the interrelationship between apnea and heart disease. For many years nasal surgeons have been studying the relationships of air movement through the nose and nasal function in an effort to diagnose and assess the effects of nasal surgery, and different nasal breathing patterns have been described as a byproduct of this testing, including an apneic pattern—the "mid cycle rest." (This was defined, essentially, as a rapid exhalation, followed by a pause lasting anywhere from a fraction of a second to as long as five seconds, after each breath.) For several years, based upon extensive clinical experience and some pilot studies, a number of rhinologists have claimed that the mid-cycle rest is associated with an increased incidence of heart disease. It is interesting to note the similarities between the two studies although the relationship needs to be studied more intensively.

In summary, then, whether making manifest the potential energy locked in nutrient food, or influencing the functional state of the cardiovascular system, or altering autonomic nervous system functioning and emotional states, the breath plays a crucial role in maintaining the integrity of the human organism. Breathing is a fundamental physiological activity which touches man's functioning on numerous levels, and as such it is a window through which these levels can be observed and manipulated. The deceptive simplicity of such a seemingly mundane process has resulted in its being overlooked in the past amidst the sophistication and complexity of our technological society. Only recently has modern Western man begun to explore some of the grosser aspects of breathing, generating a torrent of questions and speculations in the process. The results of these explorations promise to be of great practical value in understanding and modifying disease processes.

Three
Nasal Function and Energy

Rudolph Ballentine, M.D.

For some reason people don't pay much attention to the nose. Except for the cosmetic effects of its shape, it is usually regarded as little more than an opening through which air enters. If that were its sole purpose, however, one might suppose that it would be constructed differently; it should be wide and open. But the nose is actually the narrowest place in the respiratory tract. It is where the most resistance is. In other words, it is like a bottleneck; it is the one place where the air flow is most constricted as the air goes into the lungs. If you compare the work required to pull the air in and out of the nose, it is 150% of what it would be to move the air through the mouth. This is quite a difference, and it exists even when your nose is not stuffed up, but open. When one stops to consider that we breathe eighteen to twenty thousand times a day, he can begin to appreciate the amount of extra work done in twenty-four hours simply to get the air in and out the nose instead of the mouth. This uses a great deal of energy, so there must be a very good reason for doing it.

There are several good reasons. The nose does much more than simply let the air in. Medical specialists who have studied diseases of the nose (rhinologists) can list nearly thirty distinct functions that it performs. It filters, moisturizes, directs the air flow, warms the air, registers the sense of smell, brings in oxygen, creates mucus, provides a route of drainage for the sinuses, and affects the nervous system. It has a number of other functions, too, but these are the best understood.

Anatomy and Physiology of the Nose:
The word *nose* is actually a somewhat ambiguous term. To the average person it means what is visible on the face. But to physicians and physiologists it also means a mysterious and complex internal passageway that somehow involves the sinuses and the sense of smell. For this reason it is perhaps more accurate to think of there being two distinct divisions of the nose: the external and the internal. Man is unique, in terms of the external nose, for animals have no "nose" in this sense. While they have internal passageways which are often very intricate and serve a variety of important purposes, man is alone in having this peculiar protuberance on his face. Other animals have only simple openings, or holes, through which the air enters the internal nasal cavity. Even our closest relative, for example, the ape, doesn't really have a nose. While there are two nostrils, the profile of an ape shows nothing so prominent as the structure we sport. The shape of the external nose, however, plays an important role in preparing air for inhalation. This is why people who originated in different climates have different shaped noses. A long, big nose that heats the air before it gets inside is characteristic of those who live in cooler climates and also of those who live in climates, such as the Middle East, where the air is very dry. A warm, moist climate,

on the other hand, requires much less processing of the air, and the wide open nostrils of the inhabitants of tropical jungles are well known.

The external nose also serves to gather the air and accelerate its flow, forming a rapid jet that enters the cavity within the face, the internal nose. As we shall see later, the way that the stream of air is aimed inside the head can be of extreme importance. There are two parts to the external nose. One part is bone. If one feels the base of the nose he will find it to be quite hard and rigid. Moving outward, one encounters a softer area. This is made of cartilage. The first little compartment in the external nose is called the vestibule, and it is formed primarily by the two wings, or alae, of the nose which flare out on each side of it. Because they are cartilage, and relatively flexible, they tend to be influenced by gravity, so if you lie on your side the uppermost nostril will tend to be pulled downward and partially close in a valvelike way.

Moving further up the nose, there are a number of small bones and cartilages put together in an intricate way and attached to a series of bones, whose assembly is also complex, at the base of the nose. When the nose is broken it is essentially the bony parts at the root of the nose that are fractured. The flexible part, however, can also be injured, particularly internally. Inside, and toward the tip of the nose, the septum, which divides the external nose into two passageways, is also made of cartilage. Further back it is bony. Either part of it can be damaged, and this may result in the familiar "deviated septum," which tends to close off one nostril and favor the other.

As we move internally we find that the nasal

passageway expands, the dimensions of the internal nose being much larger than the vestibule. The floor of the internal nose happens also to be the roof of the mouth, and it is called the palate. If one moves his tongue backwards he finds a place where suddenly the roof of the mouth becomes softer. This, the soft palate, is made up of soft tissue only without the bony palate involved, and it ends in a little teardrop-shaped organ that we call the uvula. Just as the floor of the nose is the roof of the mouth, so is the roof of the nose also the floor of the brain and of the orbits (the cavities which house the eyeballs). In other words, we are speaking of a three-story structure. The brain, eyes and optic nerves occupy the top floor, and the mouth occupies the bottom floor. In between, on the middle floor, or second story, is the nasal cavity.

That puts the internal nose in a very interesting place, since anything going on inside of it is closely related to the brain, the nervous system, the pituitary gland, (which is located in the floor of the brain) and many other strategic structures. In addition, the first cranial nerve, which is the olfactory nerve responsible for the sense of smell, enters the nasal cavity and has its nerve endings in the uppermost parts of that compartment. This means that in order to smell something we have to direct the flow of air up toward the top part of the nasal cavity. To do this we need to create a rather brisk jet of air entering the external nose. In other words, we "sniff," and this propels a rapid stream of air inward and upward which reaches the nerve endings of the olfactory nerve.

The shape of the internal nose determines the path that the air follows. What we discover when we look

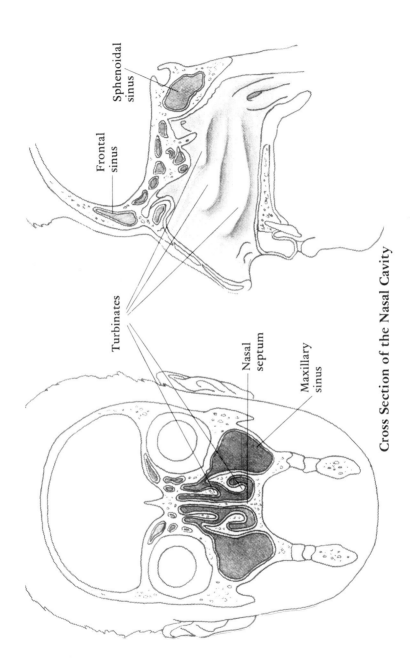

Frontal sinus

Sphenoidal sinus

Turbinates

Nasal septum

Maxillary sinus

Cross Section of the Nasal Cavity

closely inside the nasal cavity is that its walls are far from smooth. There are all sorts of strange and convoluted shapes and structures filling it, and one is prompted to conclude that the nose is some kind of junkyard where all sorts of odd organs have been thrown that didn't seem to fit anywhere else. Actually, however, it is all very intricately engineered. In fact, to really understand the nose properly one would have to be well versed in aerodynamics, for each bend and curve and nook and cranny has its purpose. Everything is cleverly designed to move the air in important directions.

The most prominent structures filling the nasal cavity are the three seashell-like bulges that one can catch a glimpse of as he looks up inside it. These are called the turbinates. As their name implies, their function is to stir and circulate the air as it enters the nose, and the result is that the stream of air passes over a much greater surface than it would otherwise. The turbinates thereby have a marked effect on the moisture content and temperature of the entering air, for as the air enters it passes over the warm, moist turbinates, picking up humidity and heat. This prepares it so that it will not be a shock to the delicate tissues of the lung.

As the air leaves the lung, the opposite reaction occurs. As it passes over the turbinates, which have just been cooled and dried by the incoming air, the outgoing air now re-warms and moistens them. In that way the turbinates help prevent the loss of heat and moisture from the body. Some animals, like the seal, have very large and complex turbinates whose surface area exceeds that of his skin. Since they live on the edge of cold, windy, salt waters, recovery of water and heat from exhaled air must be extremely important for these animals in maintaining their body temperature and conserving a salt-free internal moisture. In man, whose turbinates are much smaller, this function is apparently of less significance. In very cold weather, however, the turbinates and external nose are cooled enough so that as one exhales, the moisture in the warm air condenses on these colder structures much as moisture condenses on the cold window of an automobile, and one often develops a characteristic dripping. In fact, in very cold weather it is not uncommon to have an icicle form on the tip of the nose.

The turbinates serve, then, to baffle the air, to stir it up and to create a certain amount of turbulence. Too much turbulence, however, may cause difficulty in breathing, for it may become a great effort to pull air through such a torturous course (the degree of turbulence depends more on the arrangement of the turbinates and other structures than on the actual size of the passageway). Thus it is that some persons have difficulty breathing even though they have extremely large nasal passages.

The Mucus Blanket:

As the turbulent air is brought more thoroughly into contact with the surface of the turbinates and nasal lining, this also results in a more effective deposition of dust and other particles. To cope with this the inside of the nose is lined with a covering called a mucus membrane, so-named because it has the special property of being able to secrete mucus. Though nasal mucus is more often than not considered to be merely a nuisance, it actually performs a very vital function, for it picks up dust and debris and carries it out of the nose. This includes not only particles, but microbes such as bacteria, viruses, fungi and whatever else might be floating about in the air that is capable of invading the delicate tissues of the nose and growing, multiplying and creating that situation we call *infection*. So the mucus cannot be allowed to build up, dry out and accumulate. Some provision must be made for its removal, and the system evolved is ingenious and fascinating: Since one cannot simply lift out the nasal air filter and replace it every five thousand miles, there must be some self-cleaning mechanism in the nose so that the debris which is deposited can constantly be removed instead of accumulating. The mucus accomplishes this by constantly moving. Obviously, this is due to more than gravity. Otherwise one's nose would always be dripping, and normally the mucus does not run out of one's nostrils. In fact, it often moves against gravity, moving upward and backward, across the nasal cavity walls and towards the throat where it is swallowed and enters the esophagus. This thin coating of mucus is continuously in motion, and the result is a sort of "mucus blanket" which moves along, carrying everything with it.

The mysterious movement of this blanket is due in fact to millions of tiny hairlike structures which grow out of the mucus membrane. Called *cilia*, their untiring and consistent and continual motion is one of the miraculous phenomena of biology. That tiny subcellular structures, driven by a very simple mechanism, can manage to continually move without rest, twenty-four hours a day is no mean feat, to say the least. Moreover, their movement is coordinated; each of them works in concert with the others. Because there are so many of them, the blanket of mucus is passed over the cilia like someone handed arm-over-arm above the heads of a crowd. Thus the mucus blanket is continuously in motion, and as a result, any microbes caught up in the mucus blanket are kept moving fast enough so that they never have an opportunity to get a foothold. They can't settle in; before they get a chance to do so they are moved along. Eventually this mucus ends up in the intestinal tract where the digestive enzymes dissolve both it and the microbes it carries.

This is a beautiful system as long as it works. Unfortunately, it sometimes doesn't work. What makes it break down? If the mucus is too viscous or thick, then it very easily dries out and adheres to the cilia and mucus membrane, and at that point crusts will build up and microbes begin to invade. This is often the beginning of a cold.

The opposite extreme can also be problematic. If the mucus is too liquid, too runny, then it drips down around the cilia, and they can't keep it together and move it as an intact coating, or continuous "blanket." The result is that one develops a watery nasal drip. Again, the mucus blanket has become ineffective in protecting against infection, and when it is in this condition inflammation can easily begin. This is a frequent component of hayfever. For such reasons the consistency of the mucus is very important; as long as it is of the correct composition and viscosity, everything goes fine.

One of the primary factors determining the composition of mucus is diet. Too much starchy food as well as milk products, for instance, are notorious for creating a thicker and more viscous mucus.* In the East this is explained by defining mucus not only as a secretion, but also as an excretion. A secretion is something manufactured by the body to serve a definite purpose that is constructive; an excretion, by contrast, is something of which we are ridding ourselves. Normally, mucus is primarily a secretion. It becomes an excretion when some other excretory function of the body is not performing up to par. That is to say, mucus becomes an excretion when the lungs, the skin, the bowels, kidneys and menses are unable to rid the body of wastes that have accumulated, and mucus production increases and begins to take over some of this function.

Constipation is common in our culture. We often use antiperspirants to prevent the skin from taking its share of the excretory load. Even our breathing which, when properly regulated, can help rid the body of certain volatile wastes, is often shallow and fails to serve this purpose. To make the situation worse, since our diet often includes many processed (and therefore injured and damaged) foods, we have more of a load of wastes to get rid of in the first place, and with many of our excretory channels obstructed we are often desperate to unload from the body an accumulation of useless material. The result is often only offensive body odor or bad breath, but eventually a crisis may be reached, and the body seizes the opportunity to discharge quantities of mucus. This is

---

* For a more complete treatment of this subject see Rudolph Ballentine, M.D., *Diet and Nutrition* (Honesdale, PA: The Himalayan Institute), 1978, Ch. 10, 12.

the familiar "cold" that comes on the heels of overeating, a bad diet, or constipation. (In another era grandmother was quick to recommend a laxative at the first signs of a cold in order to prevent its developing into something severe.)

Normally the mucus and mucus membranes function in a very neat, tidy and orderly way. But when we force them to do so, they become accessory routes of excretion. Then the composition of the mucus is no longer determined by what is ideal in terms of its protective function. Rather, it is determined by what needs to be thrown off, and it becomes either too liquid, or too thick, or otherwise abnormal. The result is not only the discharge of quantities of mucus, but also the absence of the effective protection by the mucus membranes, with subsequent irritation, inflammation and often infection. Fortunately, such infection is seldom severe; it is apparently regarded by the body as a lesser evil than the retention of large quantities of useless and encumbering wastes.

This helps us to understand why dry air is sometimes so troublesome. If the mucus is already too much on the thick side, then a bit of dry air will immediately cause caking and the accumulation of crusts of mucus in the nose which, in turn, causes discomfort and irritation. This is especially true in areas where a jet of air strikes continuously. Due to the structure of the internal nose, there are certain areas where this is more likely to happen. For instance, the inflowing jet of air is reflected against the back of the nasal cavity and moves downward, striking a point at the back of the throat. Here, one is particularly likely to deposit debris, dust and microbes, and so the body has responded by stationing there a powerful concentration of lymphoid tissue which is capable of mustering white blood cells and antibodies to fight any threatening invaders. This accumulation of lymphoid tissues, though, sometimes becomes quite large and can then become a problem, with the result that the "tonsil," as the structure is called, is sometimes surgically removed to prevent its obstructing the throat. There is a growing suspicion among physicians, however, that some purposeful and valuable tissue is lost in the process, and the operation of tonsilectomy has become progressively unpopular in recent years.

Another frequent problem in the area of the nasal cavity is sinusitis. The sinuses are cavities in the facial structure that are adjacent to, and open into, the nasal cavity, (see diagram on page 63). The largest sinuses are located above each eye and in each cheek bone. Lined with mucus membrane, the sinuses can also secrete mucus, but they should, of course, remain hollow. Though their function is not fully understood, we know that in part they lend resonance to the voice by vibrating with the vocal cords. Besides the two main parts of sinuses, there are others deeper in the head, behind the nose, up under the brain and behind the eyes. These are smaller than the main sinuses, however, and less likely to cause trouble, though sometimes they can also become painful and inflamed.

Tiny passageways lead from each sinus down into the nasal cavity, and it is through these tiny passageways that the sinuses are able to drain and rid themselves of their own mucus blanket. Inflammation and problems in the sinuses result when one of the tiny passageways becomes obstructed, or clogged up, and the sinus cannot maintain a free circulation of air and mucus between itself and the nasal cavity. Normally, air moves in and out of the sinus as the stream of air flows through the nasal cavity, but when the passageway from the sinus into the nose becomes obstructed, this air flow stops, and the mucus membranes lining the sinus begin to absorb the air. This creates a kind of partial vacuum inside the sinus, and the result is to pull not only mucus, but even blood and tissue fluids, into the sinus, creating a severe irritation, pressure and pain. Then there follows what we call *sinusitis* and sometimes *sinus headache*.

The little passageways leading from the sinuses into the nasal cavity generally enter underneath the turbinates, and when these areas collect mucus that is dried or crusted, it may obstruct the passageways to the sinuses and provoke such sinus problems. One way to prevent, and gradually eliminate, such problems is the systematic use of a technique called "the nasal wash," or *neti*. This involves pouring a warm, mildly salty solution of water into one nostril and allowing it to flow out of the other. This dissolves and washes away mucus and allows the mucus membrane to function properly again. It also often frees the openings of the passageways through which the sinuses drain. Many people recoil at the idea of pouring water into the nose, but if one studies nasal function in detail, he will discover that this is far from an unnatural procedure. Actually, it is natural to have salt water inside the nose since it is not only the sinuses which empty into the internal nose, but the lacrimal duct as well.

Tears, which are salty, are produced by the lacrimal glands under the upper eyelid. They course down across the surface of the eye, keeping it moist, and are picked up by a tiny little duct in the inner, lower corner of the eye. The tears are then carried by this duct into the nasal passage where they drain along with the sinuses. When one weeps, and large amounts of tears are produced, the nose begins to "run," prompting one to reach, in the midst of an emotional scene, for a handkerchief. Even without emotion, however, tears are constantly flowing across the eye (though in smaller quantities) and constantly entering the little tunnel which carries them to the inside of the nose. In other words, one has already a continuous input of salty water into the nose at all times. Salt water is, in fact, the natural "wash" for the linings of the nasal cavity.

To capitalize on this fact, the nasal wash should be done with water that is of the same composition as tears. It should be exactly that salty, and it should be at body temperature. When done this way the nasal wash is soothing and does not irritate the linings of the nose. Iodized salt, chlorinated and chemicalized water are unnatural and may be irritating.

Nasal Wash Instructions:

Practice with a neti pot cleanses and restores health to the internal sinus passages. In yoga, breathing freely through both nostrils is also said to aid in harmonizing the active and passive systems of the body, and so the neti wash has been found to be a helpful practice before

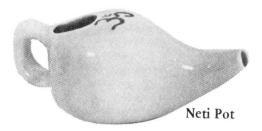

Neti Pot

meditation.

Mix well approximately one-quarter teaspoon of salt and lukewarm water in your neti pot. (The amount of salt may vary slightly with each person.) Bring the spout to the nose, and bend forward over the sink, with the head tilted to the side and slightly forward. As the water flows through the upper nostril, make slight adjustments with your head and the neti pot, if necessary, to allow the water to flow out of the other nostril.

After the pot empties, blow freely into the sink through both nostrils to clear the nose of excess water and mucus. Do not close off one nostril when doing this as it could force the water back into the ear. If there are any further problems in clearing the nostrils, kneel down and bring your forehead to the floor, raising the hips above the level of the head. Blow freely through the nostrils as before. It may also aid to turn the head to either side when doing this.

Having completed the neti wash through the nostrils in one direction, repeat the same steps on the opposite side.

After some proficiency is gained in this method, one may also learn to direct the water from the nose out through the mouth, again by making slight adjustments with the position of the head and the neti pot, and using the back of the mouth to draw the water in for spitting it out. This method is also very helpful for cleansing and ridding the nasal passages of excess mucus and dirt and restoring health to the sinus membranes.

A mucus membrane also lines the passageways that carry the air down into the lungs and chest, for the bronchi are fitted with the same kind of lining as is the nose, which secretes mucus to keep the passages moist. Otherwise the air would dry and injure them. The mucus secreted in these passageways is moved by the cilia upwards, all the way to the throat, day and night. During the day the cilia ordinarily have to work against gravity, but at night, when one lies down, their work is easier since they don't have to push the mucus uphill. For this reason, at night a great deal more mucus comes up to the throat, is cleared and swallowed. That process goes on without ceasing.

Normally, the mucus entering the gastrointestinal tract is dissolved by the juices which also kill all the microbes. This is a sort of internal ecological system in which mucus is broken down and recycled, and there is no problem. However, problems will develop as soon as mucus is excessive or when digestive juices are not present. Unfortunately, the intestinal tract tends to quiet down and rest during the night, for digestion is a process that is not normally active at this time and less digestive juice is secreted. Therefore, if the mucus is in excess, one has a stomach full of it by morning. For this reason many people wake up feeling quite uncomfortable until they eat something, which serves to either dilute the mucus or push it out of the stomach. This is especially true of people with such problems as lung diseases, emphysema, asthma, who tend to produce a great deal of mucus.

For such persons a morning wash is often recommended. Here, a large quantity of saline solution is swallowed, then thrown up. This brings out the mucus from the stomach—a simple but sound hygienic principle. The technique is called *gaj karni*, or *the upper wash*, and most well-trained yoga instructors are able to instruct one in its use.

Smokers, especially, tend to develop a great deal of mucus. A lot of this is mobilized and thrown out if they stop smoking, and after this cleansing period the lungs begin to recover. The accumulation of mucus in smokers (which creates their characteristic rattling cough and their inability to bring out the mucus that accumulates) is due to both the irritation caused by the smoke and the coal tar and to the destruction of cilia. For some reason the contents of cigarette smoke totally decimate the cilia in the mucus membranes, and this means that there is no mechanism for bringing the mucus back up out of the lungs to the throat. So it accumulates. After one stops smoking the cilia gradually begin to regenerate, and the mucus can be handled normally again.

Laterality:

If we return to the nose for a moment and look at the lining of it, we discover that underneath the mucus membrane layer is another, much thicker, layer of tissue that is spongy and can fill with large quantities of blood. This is called "erectile" tissue, and it is found only in a few areas of the body: the genitals, the breasts and the lining of the nose. Within this tissue are tiny microscopic passageways that receive blood, causing the tissue to expand, and this engorgement is the basis of erection in the genital organs (the penis or the clitoris), and there is a close relationship between these organs and the lining of the nose. In fact, this is the basis of a syndrome, familiar to ear, nose and throat doctors, which often occurs with newly-married couples. Just after marriage, during a period of continual sexual stimulation, the lining of the nose becomes chronically engorged and clogged up through a sympathetic kind of interaction. This is called *honeymoon nose.*

Sigmund Freud, in his pioneering work with sexuality, was very conscious of the interaction between the sexual organs and the nose. In fact, he originally developed his basic psychoanalytic theory through a correspondence with Wilhelm Fliess, an ear, nose and throat specialist, and the interest which drew them together was the reflexes that exist between nasal lining and reproductive organs. One of Freud's earliest theories, developed in conjunction with Fliess, was that there is a "nasal reflex neurosis." Though he later lost interest in this phenomenon, other physicians went on to elaborate on the research and to discover many interesting interrelationships. It was found, for example, that menstrual cramps were often related to an inflammation and discoloration of certain specific areas in the lining of the nose. When these were anesthetized with a small amount of topical anethetic, the menstrual pains would disappear. For some time in Germany, as a matter of fact, menstrual pain was effectively treated through cauterization, or permanent destruction, of the nerve endings in selected regions of the nose's lining.

The swelling and shrinking of the nasal erectile tissue does more, however, than simply warm the air and reflect sexual overstimulation. In fact there is a constant, regular and predictable pattern of swelling and shrinkage that the lining of the nose follows which is closely related to the whole concept of laterality in human physiology.

For instance, as the tissue covering the turbinates and the septum within one nostril swell, the tissues on the opposite side tend to become less swollen. As a result, one nostril gradually and increasingly becomes obstructed so that the flow of air is shifted to the other side. Consequently, there is a right-left dimension of breath flow: it can flow either predominantly through the right nostril or predominantly through the left nostril. If nothing is done to interfere with the rhythmic functioning of the body, this will tend to alternate in a predictable fashion. The breath will be flowing predominantly through one nostril for about an hour and forty-five minutes to two hours, after which it becomes predominant in the other side, for flow increases in one side until it reaches a peak, and then it begins to decrease. Finally, most of the air is flowing through the opposite nostril.

Though this is apparently a natural biological rhythm, it can be interfered with by emotional disturbance, irregular schedules of meals, sleep and irritation in the nose due to pollution, infection and other disrupting forces. If, however, one is healthy, tranquil, calm and living in a sensible, regular way, then the alternation of the air flow between one nostril and another follows a definite regular rhythm. This has been well documented in research laboratories both in the West and in the East.* Today this is technically called an "infradian rhythm," but its recognition is hardly a recent advance of science. In fact, it was described in great detail by the ancient yogis who, as a result of cultivating techniques of self-observation to a high degree, were able to perceive and catalogue such subtle changes in the body. Moreover, the yogis, called *swara yogis*, who focused on the science of breath made intricate correlations between the way the breath was flowing and various psychological and physiological states. They observed, for example, that having the right or left nostril open would gear us toward one activity or another in the world. If one breathes through the right side, they said, he tends to become more active and aggressive, more alert and more oriented toward the external world. Breathing through the left side, on the other hand, produces a quieter, more passive psychological state, one

* See *Science Studies Yoga*, pp. 48-50.

more oriented toward the inner world.* This is all reminiscent of what has been written recently on "right brain/ left brain," and it seems logical to ask whether right nostril flow is correlated with the predominance of one hemisphere over another. In fact, research work is in progress to answer this question.

The distinction between right and left nostril breathing, however, is more than psychological. It is said that the flow of air through the right nostril gears the internal organs toward more active *physiological* processes, too, processes such as digesting food, for example. Therefore, students of *swara yoga* were careful to open the right nostril before eating. Drinking water, by contrast, is a more passive kind of intake, and fluids were customarily taken with the left nostril open. Since they considered the side through which the air was flowing to be extremely important, the breath was attuned properly before any particular activity was undertaken. This was thought to gear both the body and the mind, preparing one mentally, emotionally and physiologically for a particular activity.

The science of breath was well known to the ancient people of India. They practiced it consistently and as a matter of course. Today, however, since most people have not developed an awareness of breath, the practices currently taught as a part of yoga are designed to help one become more sensitive to and conscious of the flow

* For further information on this difference between right and left nostril breathing and how it relates to various dichotomies in psychology and physiology such as masculinity, femininity, activity, passivity, see *Yoga and Psychotherapy*, Ch. II.

of air and what it is doing at any given moment. Such breathing exercises can also help one restore regularity, rhythm and balance to the nostril alternation.

The most commonly used of these yoga breathing exercises is called *nadi shodhanam* (alternate nostril breathing), a technique in which one deliberately changes the flow of air from one side to the other, regularly and rhythmically, through exerting pressure on the valve or lateral wall of one nostril or the other. To perform this properly, diaphragmatic breathing should have already been mastered so that the flow of air is smooth, even, consistent and well regulated.

Nadi Shodhanam:

One sits straight as though for meditation, in whatever position is comfortable, but with the head, neck and trunk relatively erect. Usually the thumb of the right hand is used to close off the right nostril while the ring finger of the same hand is used to close off the left nostril. If one finds it helpful, one can brace the hand by placing the index and middle fingers on the bridge of the nose between the eyes (if that is not found to be a distraction).

First, one exhales through the active nostril—the one that is most open. Then he inhales through the same nostril. At the end of the inhalation that nostril is closed off with the finger, allowing the exhalation to begin on the other side. At the end of that exhalation, inhalation is carried out through the same nostril, and the process is begun again. This alternation should be repeated three times so that a complete cycle is done through each nostril three times, for a total of six breaths. This is ordinarily called a "round." Customarily, a second, and then a third such round is performed so that one has breathed a total of nine inhalations and nine exhalations through each nostril. Between rounds one ordinarily takes three breaths through both nostrils.

In doing the exercise one should remember to (1) breathe slowly and gently, not so slowly that one feels that it is a strain or that he is going to run out of breath, but gently and gradually; (2) there should be no sound made by the breath. If the breath is allowed to flow gently and smoothly then less turbulence is created, and no sound vibration should result. To accomplish these two goals one must concentrate completely on the breathing itself. If the mind is allowed to wander to other subjects during the process the breathing will become irregular, jerky, noisy or otherwise disruptive. It is also important that one remain relaxed and calm during the exercise.

This is only one of three variants. The others involve exhalation through one side with inhalation through the other, and as a third variant, three complete cycles through one nostril before changing to the other side. Some students choose to do one variant for the full three rounds, while other people do a round of each variant. Consistency is probably helpful, and the variant described in the text is quite suitable for the beginner to use exclusively.

One learns through the practice of this technique to appreciate the difference between the experience of breathing through one side and breathing through the other, and he learns to increase his awareness of the nature of laterality. *Nadi shodhanam* is a study rather than simply a mechanical exercise. It is both educational and coordinating, helping to restore coordination between the two sides of the body as well as to bring back into awareness a dimension of existence which has been forgotten. We would be most embarrassed to admit that we didn't appreciate the difference between lifting the left arm and the right arm, but most persons, when asked, cannot say which nostril they're breathing through at the moment. If it is true that the right side activates a whole set of psychological and physiological functions and the left side brings into play a different set, then it would certainly be valuable to have access to an awareness of which nostril is flowing at any given moment.

The importance of this becomes especially obvious when we discover that there are techniques by means of which one can voluntarily change the flow of air from one side to the other. For example, if I lie on my left side, then the right nostril will open. It was long thought that this was because gravity pulled the blood into the lower nostril, engorging the lining, causing the turbinates to swell and closing off the "down" side. More recently, research has demonstrated that it is not actually gravity which is responsible for this shift, rather it is the pressure exerted between the down arm and the side of the chest on which one is lying. This apparently sets up a reflex which automatically dilates the nostril that is up and closes off the one which is lower, on the side where the pressure is. In any case, if I stay on one side for awhile, the opposite nostril will open. It is for this reason that the yoga manuals recommend that one lie on the left side after meals, opening the right nostril and stimulating the digestive process. Traditionally, too, it is said that when one goes to bed one should lie on the left side for five or ten minutes, activating the right nostril to create increased body heat. As soon as one is warm and comfortable he turns to the right, allowing the left nostril to open. This relaxes, calms and prepares one for sleep.

While a rhythmic alternation of air flow between one side and the other is considered natural and healthy, the persistent closure of one nostril and flow of air through the other for more than a few hours is thought to be harbinger of disease. If the breath stays in one side for six or eight hours, some illness is thought to be on its way, and if the condition lasts for a day or more the situation is said to be grave. The breath is thought to be related to the flow of energy, or *prana*, in the psychophysiological totality whose imbalances are seen as preceding the outward manifestation of disease.

Shaping the Air Currents:

While we have discussed and looked at the structure and shape of the nose and nasal cavity, there is another aspect of breathing which also has its own shape and structure. That is the air current. The pathways through which it flows, the currents and eddies and crosscurrents all make up an incredibly complex and intricate pattern of airflow that will vary from person to person, depending upon each person's nasal cavity and external nose. Just as the banks of a river shape the flow of the water, so does the nasal cavity and upper respiratory passage shape and direct the flow of air. According to the ancient yogis, this was an extremely critical issue, the flow of the air being related to the flow of energy, or *prana*, and the patterns according to which it energized body and mind.

While the yogic concepts have not been thoroughly investigated by modern research techniques, it is certainly true that many rhinologists (nose specialists) agree on the importance of the shape of the nose. Here they differ from plastic surgeons who are concerned with cosmetic effects. Their work, rather, is primarily directed toward improved functioning of the nose—that is, altering its internal structure so that misshapen passageways are restored and the air flow is corrected. Some rhinologists feel that this has an incredible impact both on the psychology and physiology of the person concerned. There are documented cases, for instance, in which the internal distortion of the nose and the abnormal flow of air so affected the person that he became mentally unbalanced. On the other hand, there are documented cases in which psychological disorders developed after nasal surgery. It is not uncommon for one to notice, after extensive restructuring of the inner nose through surgery, that he feels different.

The yogis would not be surprised by this, feeling strongly that the shape of the inner passageways and the shape of the flow of air that results is an important factor in molding both mental states and personality. According to the Eastern way of thinking, this movement of the air flow affects the way in which *prana* is supplied to the body and the brain, and in this way it influences emotions and mind. *Prana* is said to nourish the conscious mind and make it flow, pushing it in one direction or another.

This perspective on breathing has remained foreign to Western science. Nevertheless, nose surgeons who are skilled and accomplished work with this variable, intuitively structuring and reshaping the inner nose with sensitive and experienced hands. Such surgery is a crucial undertaking and not one to be taken lightly, for if the ancient ideas about breath are even partially true, to have the nose changed is to tamper with a very formative part of oneself. It should be done by an extremely competent and experienced person. Even setting a broken nose can be a delicate matter, and certainly nose surgery which ignores functional effects can be a disaster. A recent case (seen by the author) of a man who had had the turbinates removed because they seemed to obstruct the nasal passage illustrates this point. Postoperatively, the patient was so completely mentally confused that he found it necessary to give up his profession.

Of course the primary domain of the rhinologist, or nose surgeon, is the bony structure that underlies the shape of the nasal cavity. In order to determine whether surgery is required the rhinologist shrinks all of the erectile tissue lining the nasal cavity with sprays and topical applications, and then he does tests for air flow. If flow can be restored to normal through this technique, he assumes that no surgery is needed.

Actually, it is rare that the bony structure itself plays such a large role in shaping the air. It is rather the engorgement of the spongy erectile tissue which changes, shifts and causes the pattern of air flow to alter. As we have seen, the turbinates on one side engorge, closing off that nostril and resulting in a switch of air flow to the other side. This is not so simple as a matter of right or left, however. On each side there are three large turbinates as well as the inner surface of the septum, each of which is covered with erectile tissue. The degree and location of swelling in each of these can vary, and the permutations and combinations are incredible. The result is a complex, continually changing pattern of air flow which can only be likened to the result of driving a large, heavy-duty vehicle with three separate gear shifts, each gear shift having a number of positions, so that the resulting combinations are numerous.

From the perspective of ancient Eastern ideas about breathing the turbinates, by combining in various ways to create a varying pattern of air flow , help gear us to different activities. This is a continuously changing phenomenon, both influencing and resulting from emotional states, mental states and physiological functions. The pattern of engorgement in the turbinates and the resulting shape of air flow is apparently like a central clearing house, or switchboard, where all the body's functions are having an effect, and all the body's functions are in turn being affected. In fact, research has shown that the flow of air touching the surface of various areas of the turbinates triggers neuronal responses that set up reflexes throughout the body. In other words, a specific current of air sends out ripples into both the lungs and the nervous system, that affect the whole person. In the ancient scriptures very specific descriptions are given of various patterns of air flow and their relationship to personality states and physiological function. Laboratory research is gradually gaining the sophisticated technology needed to be able to look into and disprove or verify these ancient ideas.

Nasal Functioning and the Limbic System:

Neurophysiologists have found that inhalation not only stimulates the olfactory nerve when the air contains substances that can be sensed with the sense of smell, it also triggers neuronal messages in the olfactory nerve even when the air is clean. Why this occurs is not known. It is known, however, that the olfactory nerve and the part of the brain that it reaches is integrally connected to the limbic system, that part of the central nervous system which subserves emotional states. We all know that odors are closely connected to emotions, a fact which is put into practice every time a bit of perfume is dabbed behind the ears. To discover, however, that the same brain structures may be brought into play simply through the movement of air is intriguing.

The breath has, then, a profound effect on man's physical and psychological functioning, since it is the link between the body and mind. The nose, therefore, as the major portal of breath into the body, plays a crucial role. It prepares and modifies the breath for assimilation by the body, interacting with both the external and internal environment, changing its activity to meet the body's energy demands from moment to moment, and an awareness of the functioning of the nose lends an added dimension to both psychological and physiological self awareness.

Four

The Science of Prana

Swami Rama

The Sanskrit word, *pranayama* is usually translated as the science of breath, but this translation is a very limited interpretation of the word, for *pranayama* literally means the *ayama* (expansion or manifestation) of *prana* (*pra*: first unit; *na*: energy). Prana is the vital energy of the universe. According to one of the schools of Indian philosophy, the whole universe is derived from *akasha* (space or ether) through the energy of *prana*. *Akasha* is hence the infinite, all-encompassing material of the universe, and *prana* is the infinite, all-pervading energy of the universe—cosmic energy. All the diverse forms of this universe are sustained by the energy of *prana*, and *pranayama* is the science which imparts knowledge related to the control of *prana*. One who has learned to control *prana* has learned to control all the energies of this universe—physical and mental. He has also learned to control his body and his mind.

The mind stands as a wall between the yogi and the reality. When the student comes in touch with the finer forces called *prana* he can learn to control his mind, for it is tightly fastened to the *prana* like a kite to a string. When the string is held skillfully the kite, which wants to fly here and there, is controlled and flies in the direction desired. All breathing exercises—advanced or basic—enable the student to control his mind through understanding *prana*. Thus, the science of breath helps the student of yoga to bring *prana* under control in order to attain the higher rungs of spirituality. He who has controlled his breath and *prana* has also controlled his mind. He who has controlled his mind has also controlled his breath.

All aspects and principles that constitute the universe, or macrocosm, are embodied in all the microcosmic forms that constitute the universe—just as the mighty ocean is completely represented in a single, small drop of water from that ocean. The human body is sustained by the same *prana* that sustains the universe, and it is through the manifestation of *prana* that all body functions are possible and coordinated.

According to the ancient manuals of yoga the cosmic force of *prana* in the human body is recognized and subdivided on the basis of the ten functions it performs, and of the ten *pranas*, there are five major and five minor ones. The major *pranas* are *udana, prana, samana, apana* and *vyana*. Though the word *prana* is applied to the universal *prana* that includes all ten *pranas*, one of the five major *pranas* has also been given the name *prana*. The context of usage will enable one to differentiate between the specific and the generalized energy.

Udana rules the region of the body above the larynx and governs the use of our special senses. *Prana* rules the region between the larynx and the base of the heart. It governs speech and the vocal apparatus as well as the respiratory system and the muscles engaged in it. *Samana* rules in the region between the heart and the navel and governs all the metabolic activity engaged in digestion. *Apana* has its abode below the navel and governs the functions of the kidneys, the colon, the rectum, the bladder and the genitals. *Vyana* pervades the whole body and governs the relaxation and contraction of all muscles, voluntary and involuntary, as well as the movement of the joints and the structures around them.

The energy of *prana* is subtle in form. Its most external manifestation is the breath, and of the five major *pranas, prana* is the energy that governs the breath. Then, through control of respiration, the yogi proceeds to control of the other subtle energies of *prana*, and this may explain the use of the same word for the universal energy as well as for the specific *prana* governing respiration. The importance of this specific *prana* in allowing us access to the subtler energies of the cosmic *prana* is also seen in the fact that what we call death, that is the death of the physical body, results from the cessation of respiration.

The sequence in which one proceeds from control of the breath to control of the cosmic energy of *prana* is clearly illustrated by the following story that Swami Vivekananda tells in his book on raja yoga:

There once was a king's minister who fell into disgrace and was imprisoned at the top of a tall tower. The minister asked his faithful wife to come to the tower when darkness had fallen, bringing with her a long rope, some stout twine, string, silken thread, a beetle and some honey. Though bewildered by this strange request, the good wife did as he bade her. The minister then asked his wife to tie the silken thread to the beetle, to smear some honey on its horns and then to set it on the tower wall with its head pointed toward the top of the tower. The beetle, enticed onward by the sweet smell of the honey, slowly made its way to the top of the tower, pulling the silken thread behind it. The minister took hold of the silken thread and then asked his wife to tie the string to the other end of the silken thread. Using the silken thread he drew up the string. In like manner he used the string to draw up the stout twine, and the twine to draw up the rope. Then he descended to freedom, using the rope.

In our bodies the breath is like the silken thread, using which we skillfully grasp the string of the nerve impulses; from these we grasp the stout twine of our thoughts; and finally we grasp the rope of *prana*, thus gaining our ultimate freedom.

Pranayama and the Nervous System:

In order to understand the science of *pranayama* it is necessary to consider the nature and functions of the nervous system, for this system coordinates the functions of all the other systems in the body. Subdivided into the central and the autonomic nervous systems, the central nervous system consists of the brain, twelve pairs of cranial nerves, the spinal cord and thirty-one pairs of spinal nerves. The cranial and spinal nerves spread throughout the body, forming a network of nerve fibers; efferent, or motor nerve fibers, carry nerve impulses from the brain and spinal cord outward to the nerve endings, and afferent, or sensory nerve fibers, carry nerve impulses from the nerve endings inward to the brain and spinal cord. To illustrate the functions of the afferent and efferent fibers, consider the case of stubbing one's toe. The nerve endings at the toe send nerve impulses along the afferent fibers to the spinal cord and brain. The brain interprets these impulses as pain and reacts to the pain by sending motor impulses along the efferent fibers outward to the hands, enabling them to reach out and soothe the injured toe.

Patanjali, the codifier of yoga science, explains that the control of *prana* is the regulation of inhalation and exhalation. This is accomplished by eliminating the pause between inhalation and exhalation or expanding it by retention. Then, by regulating the motion of the lungs, the heart and the vagus nerve are controlled. The autonomic nervous system regulates processes in our bodies which are not normally under our voluntary control—processes such as secretion by the digestive organs, the beating of the heart and the movement of the lungs. The science of *pranayama* is thus intimately connected with the autonomic nervous system and brings its functions under conscious control through the functioning of the lungs. Here is a unique exception to the rule that the autonomic nervous system governs processes that are self-regulating and not under voluntary control. Though the act of respiration is for the most part involuntary, voluntary control in this area is easily achieved, for the depth, duration and frequency of respiration can be consciously modulated quite readily. It is for this reason that control of breath constitutes an obvious starting point toward attainment of control over the functioning of the autonomic nervous system.

The autonomic nervous system is subdivided into the sympathetic and the parasympathetic nervous systems. As the names indicate, these two subsystems work in seeming opposition to each other, yet the net result is harmonious regulation. The parasympathetic system, for instance, tries to slow down the heart while the sympathetic system accelerates it, and between these two opposing actions the heart rate is regulated. The sympathetic nervous system consists mainly of two vertical rows of ganglia, or nerve cell clusters, arranged on either side of the spinal column. Branches from these gangliated cords spread out to different glands and viscera in the thorax and abdomen, forming integrated plexuses with nerve branches of the parasympathetic system. The main part of this system is the tenth cranial nerve, also called the vagus, or wandering, nerve which is connected with the hindbrain and travels downwards along the spinal cord through the neck, chest and abdomen, sending out branches to form various plexuses with the sympathetic system. It ends in a plexus which is connected to the solar plexus; but even though it ends at the solar plexus, it is connected with the lower plexuses through filaments.

There are only two known ways of having conscious control over our involuntary nervous system. One is that it can be brought under conscious control by systematically practicing breathing exercises and by preparing oneself for understanding the various vehicles and channels of *prana*. But first of all one should learn to regulate the motion of the lungs so that the heart

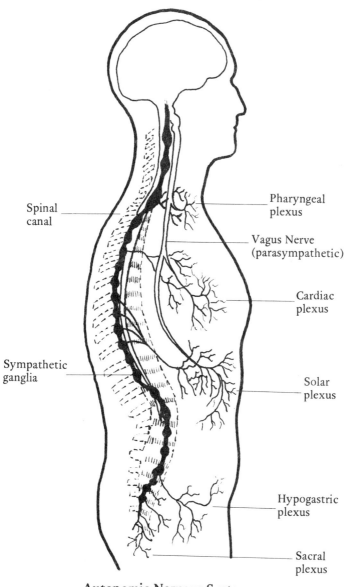

Spinal canal

Pharyngeal plexus

Vagus Nerve (parasympathetic)

Cardiac plexus

Sympathetic ganglia

Solar plexus

Hypogastric plexus

Sacral plexus

Autonomic Nervous System

function is regulated. Then the right vagus nerve is brought under conscious control, and the portion of the mind that coordinates with the involuntary system thus is accessible to the student. The other way of gaining control over the autonomic nervous system is through will power. The more the mind is dissipated, the more the will is scattered. When the mind is made one-pointed, the mind strengthens the will power, and with the help of the will power the autonomic nervous system functions in the way we want it to. Thus, it is true that there is no such thing as an involuntary system if one learns to control and regulate the motion of the lungs. For by doing so, a vast portion of that system is brought under control.

Modern scientists give importance to breathing exercises only from the viewpoint of oxygen intake, and their concern is with the absorption of oxygen in large enough quantities to vitalize the nervous system. But in the science of breath related to *pranayama*, this is a minor consideration. More detailed knowledge and experience is needed to study the finer forces of life than the mere intake of oxygen and output of carbon dioxide. The ancient manuals of yoga anatomy, for instance, describe a network of several thousand *nadis*, or channels, through which the currents of *prana* flow, energizing and sustaining all parts of the body as well as the several thousand *nadis*.

The words *nadis, channels* and *vehicles* are meant to explain one and the same force which is called *pranic* force. According to some manuals the number of *nadis* is 72,000 (other manuals talk about 350,000 *nadis*). Fourteen are more important than the others, but the most

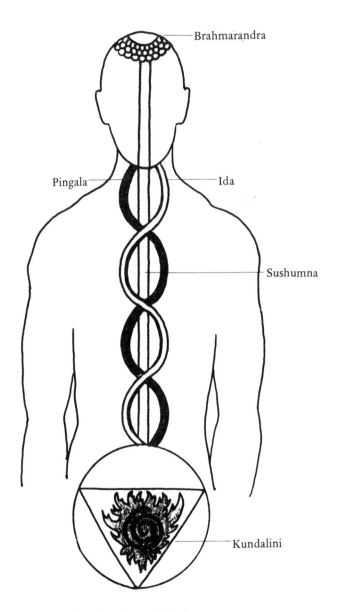

Ida, Pingala and Sushumna

important among these are six: *ida, pingala, sushumna, brahmani, chitrani,* and *vijnana.* Among these six, three are the most important: *pingala (surya)* which flows through the right nostril; *ida (chandra)* which flows through the left nostril; *sushumna,* which is a moment when both nostrils flow freely without any obstruction. Expansion of that moment is called *sandhya,* and for meditation the application of *sushumna* is of prime importance, for after applying *sushumna* the meditator cannot be disturbed by mere sounds, noises or other disturbances from the external world, nor by the bubbles of thought arising from the unconscious and going through the conscious mind during meditation

All three of the major *nadis* originate at the base of the spine and travel upwards. The *sushumna nadi* is centrally located and travels along the spinal canal. At the level of the larynx it divides into an anterior portion and a posterior portion, both of which terminate in the *brahmarandra,* or Cavity of Brahma, which corresponds to the ventricular cavity in the physical body. The *ida* and *pingala nadis* also travel upwards along the spinal column, but they crisscross each other and the *sushumna* before terminating in the left and right nostrils, respectively.

The junctions of *ida, pingala* and *sushumna* along the spinal column are called *chakras,* or wheels, and just as the spokes of a wheel radiate outward from the central hub, so do the other *nadis* radiate outward from the *chakras* to other parts of the body. In other words, the *chakras* are junctions of other *nadis* with the three main *nadis: sushuman, ida* and *pingala.*

There are seven principal *chakras*: the *muladhara chakra* at the base of the spine at the level of the pelvic plexus in the physical body, the *swadhisthana chakra* at the level of the hypogastric plexus, the *manipura chakra* at the level of the solar plexus, the *anahata chakra* at the level of the cardiac plexus, the *vishuddha chakra* at the level of the pharangeal plexus, the *ajna chakra* at the level of the nasociliary plexus and the *sahasrara chakra* at the top of the head. The anterior portion of the *sushumna* passes through the *ajna chakra* and the posterior portion passes behind the skull, the two portions uniting in the *brahmarandra*.*

Scientists have made many attempts to identify the *nadis* with what we know of modern anatomy, but they have not been able to do so. Yoga anatomy and physiology, however, is very clear and accurate to those who systematically practice and study the science of yoga, and they find that it reveals more about the internal functionings of the human body than any modern scientific experiment or explanation. It is true, however, that the ancient description of *nadis* and *chakras* bears a remarkable resemblance to modern anatomical descriptions of nerves and plexuses, respectively. Some scientists have tried to establish a correspondence between the two systems, but the assumption behind such an attempt is that the nerves and plexuses belong to the physical body while the *nadis* and *chakras* belong to what is known in yoga science as the subtle body. In other words, they are the subtle counterparts of the

*These centers are described more fully in *Yoga and Psychotherapy*, p. 216 ff.

nerves and plexuses, respectively. The currents of *prana* flowing through these *nadis* are the subtle counterparts of the nerve impulses. The yogis did not dissect the physical body in order to learn about *nadis* and *chakras* (and such a dissection of the physical body would be futile). They discovered the network of *nadis* and *chakras* by mapping the flow of *prana* through this network, and they developed this mapping ability through introspective experimentation.

The physical body is built around the subtle framework of the *nadis*, then, and the sustenance of the body is through the flow of the energy of *prana* through this network of *nadis*. In the average individual the dynamic and creative aspect of the energy of *prana* is only an infinitesimal fraction of the total energy of *prana*, the major part of it being in a potential, or seed, state. The manuals of yoga refer to this latent, stored-up energy as *kundalini*, the symbolic representation of which is that of a sleeping serpent coiled up in the *muladhara chakra* at the base of the spine. Further, in the average individual there is flow of *prana* through *ida* and *pingala*, but not through *sushumna*, this *nadi* being blocked at the base of the spinal column.

The techniques of *pranayama* are aimed at de-vitalizing *ida* and *pingala* and at the same time opening up the *sushumna nadi*, thus allowing the *prana* to flow through this channel. The yogi then experiences great joy and is freed from the bondage of time, space and causation. Then, having opened up the *sushumna nadi* the yogi rouses the sleeping serpent at the *muladhara chakra* and guides the tremendous energy thus activated

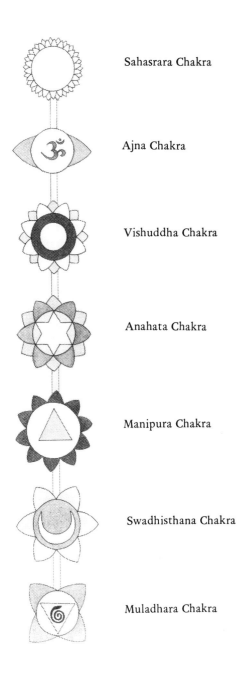

Sahasrara Chakra

Ajna Chakra

Vishuddha Chakra

Anahata Chakra

Manipura Chakra

Swadhisthana Chakra

Muladhara Chakra

upward along *sushumna*, piercing the six *chakras*, to the seventh *chakra*, called the *sahasrara chakra*, represented as a thousand-petaled lotus at the crown of the head. This arousal and ascent of the latent *kundalini* energy and its merging in the *sahasrara* is synonymous with the union of cosmic potency, or *shakti*, with cosmic consciousness, or *shiva*, and with this union the yogi achieves liberation from all miseries and bondage. He thus merges his individual soul, or *atman*, with the cosmic soul, or *Brahman*.

Pranayama is one of the rungs on the ladder of raja yoga. The first four rungs of the ladder are referred to by some as hatha yoga, or physical yoga, and the last four rungs as raja yoga or the royal yoga. The first four rungs are *yama*, or restraints, *niyama*, or observances, *asana*, or posture, and *pranayama*. The four higher rungs are *pratyahara*, or sense withdrawal, *dharana*, or concentration, *dhyana*, or meditation, and *samadhi*, the superconscious state, the ultimate freedom from the cycle of birth and death.*

Controlling the breath and calming the nerves is a prerequisite to controlling the mind, and control of the mind is a prerequisite to the ultimate subjugation of the universal energy of *prana*. To the yogi body, breath, nerves, mind, *prana* and the universe are all part of a continuum, and he does not set up artificial compartments between these various entities. In Western thinking, however, there has been a much greater tendency for such compartmentalization, and the sciences of physiology

* For more detailed information on the eight rungs of the yoga ladder see Swami Rama, *Lectures on Yoga* (Honesdale, PA: The Himalayan Institute), 1979.

and psychology have maintained their separate identities. Only in recent times have scientists admitted the inter-relationship between psyche and soma, and the psychosomatic origins of disease have thus become a valid subject for research and study.

According to yoga and the science of *pranayama*, disease is a manifestation of an imbalance in the flow of *prana* (the energy of *prana* includes both physical and mental energies, body and mind both being sustained by *prana*), and body and mind interact to a greater extent than is normally imagined. We will consider several examples of such interaction. In the stomach the food is mixed thoroughly with the digestive juices by the action of peristalsis, or muscular churning, and scientific experiments have shown that peristalsis is greatly inhibited by emotions such as anger, fear and anxiety. Another example of the interrelationship between body and mind is the influence of emotions on the breathing. When one is afraid, the breathing becomes shallow and rapid; when depressed, the breathing becomes heavy and labored.*

Psychologists have shown that there is a correspondence between personality types and breathing patterns. Yoga science also recognizes such a correspondence, but according to yoga, the relationships between the breath and the mind are reciprocal. If a certain state of mind results in a certain mode of breathing, then, conversely, by adopting that mode of breathing consciously one can evoke the corresponding state of mind.

*See *Yoga and Psychotherapy*, pp. 34-37.

If there is a correspondence between personality type and pattern of breathing, then the yogi states categorically that by changing the pattern of breathing one can transform the personality for when the mind is disturbed the breath is disturbed and becomes shallow, rapid and uneven. By consciously making the breath deep, even and regular, one will experience a noticeable release of tension and an increased sense of relaxation and tranquility.

Basic Breathing Techniques:

Respiration is the most important function of the body. It is the source of all energy and life to the living being, just as the mainspring is to a clock. Yet most people are not aware of the simple fact that the breath does not flow equally through the two nostrils. At times one nostril is more active than the other, and at other times it may become more dormant than the other.* This is because within the nose, on each side of the septum separating the two nostrils, there are structures called turbinates that regulate the pathway of the air within the inner nose. These turbinates are covered by mucus membrane, and this membrane is composed of erectile tissue. The swelling of the turbinates changes the inner configuration of the air pathways, and it can thus block or restrict the flow of air. This explains the unequal flow of breath through the nostrils. One of the aims of yogic breathing techniques is to equalize this flow, for

* For further information on the subject of nostril dominance see *Yoga and Psychotherapy*, pp. 37-42, and *Science Studies Yoga*, pp. 48-50.

such equilization is a preliminary to the devitalization of the *ida* and *pingala nadis* and the opening up of the blocked *sushumna nadi*. We will consider, later, a breathing technique called *nadi shodhanam*, or purification of the *nadis*, the practice of which will lead to equalization of the breath in the right and left nostrils and thence to the opening up of the *sushumna nadi*. Equalizing the flow of breath calms the mind, and in states of deep meditation the equal flow of breath through both nostrils is evident.

Jala Neti:

A preliminary to equalizing the flow of breath is cleansing the nostrils, and for this manuals of yoga describe a technique called *jala neti*, or purification with water. Here, lukewarm water, with a little salt dissolved in it, is poured into one nostril while the head is tilted so as to allow the salt water to flow out through the other nostril. (A cup can be used to do this, but it is far more convenient to use a pot with a narrow spout.) This lukewarm, saline water not only dissolves and washes away any accumulated mucus and dirt, but it also, by osmosis, draws out excess water from swollen turbinate structures. It also facilitates drainage of the sinuses. If the water is first poured into the left nostril and flows out through the right, the flow direction is then reversed by pouring the salt water into the right nostril and allowing it to drain through the left. This accomplishes a thorough cleansing of the air passageways. Personal instruction in this technique and demonstration from a qualified teacher is recommended. Daily practice prevents congestion of the sinuses and makes one less susceptible to common colds and other respiratory infections.

Sutra Neti—String Neti:

In this exercise a rubber catheter with a cotton string attached to it is inserted in the nostril and then taken out through the mouth, or the string alone may be used if the end has been stiffened with wax. All the implements should be sterilized before they are used and, as has been said before, the demonstration of this technique by a competent teacher is recommended.

This exercise cleanses the nostrils, strengthens the mucus membrane and is beneficial for the eyes.

Rhythmic Diaphragmatic Breathing:

The most important aspect of breathing is diaphragmatic breathing. The average person uses his chest muscles rather than his diaphragm when he breathes, and such breathing is usually shallow, rapid and irregular. As a consequence the lower lobes of the lungs, which receive an abundant supply of blood, are not adequately ventilated, and the gas exchange which takes place between the air in the lungs and the blood is inadequate. Respiratory physiologists refer to this as a ventilation-perfusion abnormality. With diaphragmatic breathing such inequalities between ventilation and perfusion are minimized. There is also evidence to suggest that diaphragmatic breathing is beneficial because it increases the suction pressure created in the thoracic cavity and improves the venous return of blood, thereby reducing the load on the heart and enhancing circulatory function.

Though chest breathing has now become natural and involuntary for most of us, it is really a part of the fight/flight syndrome, aroused when the organism is challenged by some external stress or danger. Because of the reciprocity between breath and mind, chest breathing, in turn, gives rise to the tension and anxiety associated with the fight/flight syndrome. With chest breathing, the breath is shallow, jerky and unsteady, resulting in similar unsteadiness of the mind. All techniques aimed at providing relaxation of the body, nerves and mind will be ineffective unless chest breathing is replaced by deep, even and steady diaphragmatic breathing.

Although diaphragmatic breathing is very simple, easy and beneficial, the habit of doing it has to be consciously cultivated before it can become automatic. A simple practice to achieve this is to lie down on one's back on a mat or rug, with one palm placed on the center of the chest and the other on the lower edge of the rib cage where the abdomen begins. As one inhales, the lower edge of the rib cage should expand and the abdomen should rise; as one exhales the opposite should occur; there should be relatively little movement of the upper chest. By practicing diaphragmatic breathing one finds in due time that this exercise is becoming habitual and automatic.

Next one should cultivate the habit of harmonious, rhythmic breathing along with diaphragmatic breathing (observing the rate of breathing per minute on both inhalation and exhalation is highly therapeutic and is not at all difficult). Breathing between sixteen and twenty breaths per minute is considered average, but when both inhalation and exhalation become slower and smoother breathing becomes very easy. The student should learn to slow down his inhalation first because inhalation is affected by nerve centers, the diaphragm, the intercostal and abdominal muscles. What is more, modern scientists are aware that during inhalation plasma from the capillaries oozes out into the alveolar space (it returns again into the circulation during exhalation). During inhalation nutrients from the blood ooze out into the air sacs (there is an ample supply of enzymes within the sacs to act on the nutrient materials which contain protein, fatty acids and carbohydrates), so lengthening the inspiration increases the time for the metabolic function to take place within the air sacs.

Rhythmic diaphragmatic breathing also brings more air and oxygen into the air sacs of the lungs and into the blood stream. It increases the return of venous blood to the lungs and sends an increased blood supply to the capillaries of the alveoli. It can be practiced in a firm standing position, a steady sitting position, or by lying on one's back with the hands along the sides of the body, palms upward, and legs slightly apart (this latter posture is called *shavasana,* or the corpse posture).* Exhalation should be through the nostrils, and there should be no external sound. Having exhaled completely, inhalation begins, minimizing the pause, again using the nostrils and making no external sound.

* See *Science Studies Yoga,* pp. 50-53.

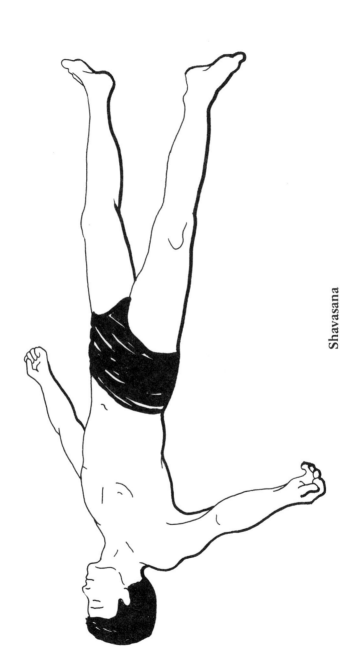

Shavasana

Makarasana or Crocodile:

Those who do not understand and, for some reason, cannot start practicing diaphragmatic breathing in a sitting position should place themselves in the crocodile posture.* Lie on the stomach, placing the legs a comfortable distance apart and pointing the toes outward. Fold the arms in front of the body, resting the hands on the biceps. Position the arms so that the chest does not touch the floor. This not only necessitates diaphragmatic breathing, it also teaches one how it feels to breathe diaphragmatically, for when one inhales he feels the abdomen pressed against the floor, and when he exhales he feels the abdominal muscles relaxing. So one can easily notice the movement of the diaphragm when he is in this posture.

Sandbag Breathing:

A bag containing between ten and fifteen pounds of sand is placed between the chest and abdomen of a normal person. After closing the teeth, sealing the lips gently, and lying on the back in *shavasana*, one can practice diaphragmatic breathing without any effort. This exercise strengthens the diaphragm.

Diaphragmatic breathing decreases the breath rate considerably. It is the basic exercise that the student practices to accomplish the higher practices and derive benefits from the science of breath and *pranayama*.

---

* See Samskrti and Veda, *Hatha Yoga Manual One* (Honesdale, PA: The Himalayan Institute), 1979, pp. 64-65.

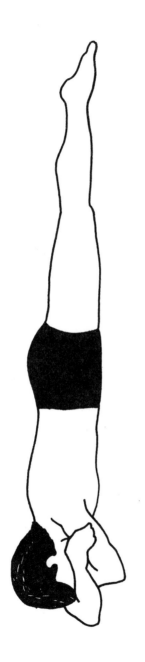

Makarasana, or Crocodile Posture

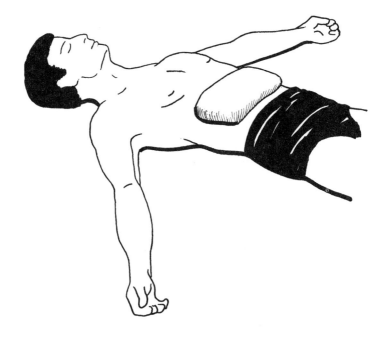

Sandbag Breathing

Breathing air into the deep recesses of the lungs is healthy in all respects. Since the pericardium is attached to the diaphragm, the process of deep breathing causes the daiphragm to descend, stretching the heart downward toward the abdomen. When the lungs are filled with air from the bottom upwards, they compress, giving a gentle massage to the heart. As the diaphragm contracts and relaxes, it also massages the heart, liver and pancreas and helps to improve the functions of the spleen, stomach, small intestine and abdomen as well.

If the practice of rhythmic diaphragmatic breathing is done ten times a day for at least two months, with gradual and equal prolongation of the inhalation and exhalation, the body will experience a sense of deep relaxation and rest—more restful even than the deepest sleep. One will remain free from the stress and strain which is the source of many physical and psychosomatic illnesses. The nerves will be calm, and the voice and face will manifest this calmness. The voice will grow sweeter, and the harsh lines of the face will be replaced by a soft glow.

Nadi Shodhanam:

Another excellent breathing exercise is called *nadi shodhanam* or channel purification.

1) Sit in a calm, quiet, airy place in an easy and steady posture with the head, neck and trunk erect and in a straight line. The body should be still.

2) Bring the right hand up to the nose; the index and middle fingers should be folded so that the right thumb

can be used to close the right nostril and the ring finger used to close the left nostril (*vishnu mudra*).

3) With the right nostril closed, and using the right thumb, exhale completely through the left nostril. The exhalation should be slow, controlled and free from exertion and jerkiness.

4) At the end of the exhalation close the left nostril with the ring finger, open the right nostril and inhale slowly and completely. Inhalation should also be slow, smooth, controlled and of the same duration as exhalation.

5) Repeat this cycle of exhalation through the left nostril followed by inhalation through the right nostril two more times.

6) At the end of the third inhalation through the right nostril, exhale completely through the same nostril, still keeping the left nostril closed with the ring finger.

7) At the end of this exhalation close the right nostril and inhale through the left nostril. Repeat two more times. This completes the exercise.

In summary, the exercise consists of:

a) Three cycles of exhalation through the left nostril and inhalation through the right nostril, followed by

b) Three cycles of exhalation through the right nostril and inhalation through the left nostril.

In the evening start the exercise with three cycles of exhalation through the right nostril and inhalation through the left nostril followed by three cycles of exhalation through the left nostril and inhalation through the right nostril. In all phases of this exercise the exhalation and inhalation should be of equal duration, without a pause between exhalation and inhalation. Breathing should be diaphragmatic and should be slow and controlled, with no sense of exertion. With practice, gradual lengthening of the duration of inhalation and exhalation should be attempted.

There are slight variations on this basic technique in different yoga texts. One should avoid confusion and frequent changes in technique, however, for only with regular practice of the same technique can one reap the full benefits of *nadi shodhanam*. Further, in some texts retention of the breath between inhalation and exhalation is recommended. This is an advanced form of the exercise and should be attempted only under the guidance of a competent teacher. Otherwise the student may harm himself irreparably. Under proper guidance retention may be practiced, the period of retention being gradually increased so long as it does not in any way affect the rhythm, evenness and equality of inhalation and exhalation. The recommended ratio between the durations of inhalation, retention and exhalation is 1:4:2. After mastering the retention of breath after inhalation, one attempts retention after exhalation, again with gradual lengthening of the duration of retention.

Pranayama is a highly developed and complex science, and the advanced techniques require expert guidance. They should not be attempted purely on the basis of instructions found in books. Unless one has the prerequisites for such advanced techniques more harm than good will ensue, for the aspirant will have awakened the energies of *prana* to a degree that is beyond his capacity to contain and control.

The basic form of *nadi shodhanam* without retention, described above, and a few other types of *pranayama* may be practiced safely, based on the instructions given here. But to repeat: retention of breath does require the sanction and guidance of a teacher well versed in *pranayama*.

Kapalabhati Pranayama:

In literal translation this means, "the *pranayama* that makes the forehead and entire face lustrous." It helps clean the sinuses and all other respiratory passages and stimulates the abdominal muscles and digestive organs. A sense of exhilaration is experienced with this practice.

This exercise consists of a vigorous and forceful expulsion of breath, using the diaphragm and abdominal muscles, followed by a relaxation of the abdominal muscles resulting in a slow, passive inhalation. This cycle of an active and vigorous exhalation followed by a passive inhalation is repeated several times in quick succession. In the beginning one attempts between seven and twenty-one cycles, depending on one's capacity.

Bhastrika Pranayama:

The word *bhastrika* means, "bellows," and in this *pranayama* the abdominal muscles work like bellows. The beneficial effects of this exercise are similar to those of *kapalabhati*.

In this exercise, the diaphragm and abdominal muscles are employed, as in *kapalabhati*, but here both inhalation and exhalation are vigorous and forceful. Between seven and twenty-one cycles may be attempted, according to one's capacity, and the cycles should follow each other in quick succession.

Ujjayi Pranayama:

The word *ujjayi* may be interpreted as, "control or victory arising from a process of expansion." This *pranayama* enhances the ventilation of the lungs, removes phlegm, calms the nerves and fills the whole body with vitality.

Inhalation and exhalation during *ujjayi* are slow and deep, and take place with partial closure of the glottis. This produces a sound like sobbing, but it is even and continuous. During inhalation the incoming air is felt on the roof of the palate and is accompanied by the sibilant sound *sa*. During exhalation the outgoing air is felt on the roof of the palate and is accompanied by the aspirate sound *ha*. During inhalation the abdominal muscles are kept slightly contracted, and during exhalation abdominal pressure is exerted till the breath is completely expelled.

Bhramari Pranayama:

Bhramari is a large bee, and the sound of a bee is made during exhalation in this exercise. Inhale completely through both nostrils. Exhaling, as in *ujjayi*, produce the humming sound of a bee. Repeat for two to three minutes. *Bhramari* soothes the nerves and calms the mind.

Sitali Pranayama:

Sitali and *sitkari* both are exercises for cooling and soothing the body. Curl the tongue lengthwise until it resembles a tube (those students who cannot do this should practice *sitkari*). Let the tip of the tongue protrude outside the lips. Inhaling, make a hissing sound with the breath. Exhale completely through both nostrils. Repeat three times.

Sitkari Pranayama:

Roll the tongue back as far as possible toward the soft palate. Let the lips part, and clench the teeth. Inhaling through the teeth, make a hissing sound with the breath. Exhale completely through both nostrils. Repeat three times.

The following exercises (*suryabhedana, murccha* and *plavini*) are studied only under a teacher. They are never learned, and should not be practiced, from a manual.

Suryabhedana Pranayama:

In this exercise the breath is inhaled through the right nostril, retained, and then exhaled through the left nostril.

Murccha Pranayama:

Inhale completely through both nostrils. Apply the chin lock, and then slowly and gently exhale.

Plavini Pranayama:

Plavini is one of the most advanced *pranayama* exercises. Here the stomach is first filled completely with air. Then, while the air remains in the stomach, the lungs are filled completely. The breath is retained, and then finally exhaled. This method of inhalation, retention and exhalation is repeated the desired number of times, and when the exercise is finished the air is regurgitated through the mouth.

There are a few, more rare, advanced *pranayama* exercises which are meant exclusively for the adept yogis. Such exercises are traditionally imparted to the advanced students by their preceptors.

Patanjali, the codifier of the Yoga Sutras, while explaining various ways and methods of bringing the mind under control, also includes the method of *pranayama*. The whole secret of the science of breath lies in the interpretation of Sutra 1:34. Here Patanjali uses different words for inhalation, exhalation and retention. According to him, having control over the pause is called *pranayama*. This means that to control, eliminate and expand the pause is *pranayama*. In Sanskrit the pause is called *kumbhaka*. Hence, it is an aphorism; it is like a brief note that is meant for the competent teacher to explain to his students. Actually, *pranayama*, in practice means *pause*, though various authors have tried to explain it in various ways. All the breathing exercises in practice are meant to control, eliminate and expand that pause; thus *pranayama* means *a pause*.

Hatha yoga manuals mention eight varieties of *kumbhaka*. It is a practical subject, and competent yogis alone know the secrets of the nature of the pause. The *kumbhakas* should be practiced carefully under a competent guide, never by reading manuals alone. Nor should they be practiced without applying the *bandhas*.

Bandhas and Their Application:

All aspirants are strictly advised not to practice the exercises of *kumbhaka*, or retention of breath, without applying the *bandhas*. *Bandhas* are locks, and there are three of them: *jalandhara bandha*, the chin lock; *uddiyana bandha*, the abdominal lock; and *mulabandha*, the anal lock.

Jalandhara Bandha:

The internal and external carotid arteries, which bring the blood supply to the brain, lie on both sides of the neck. When conscious pressure is applied to these arteries through the chin lock, *jalandhara bandha*, the nerve impulses traveling to the brain fade the body consciousness and bring about a trancelike condition. This stimulation also slows down the heart, and the *vijnani nadi*, which can be translated as "channel of consciousness," can thus be brought under conscious control.

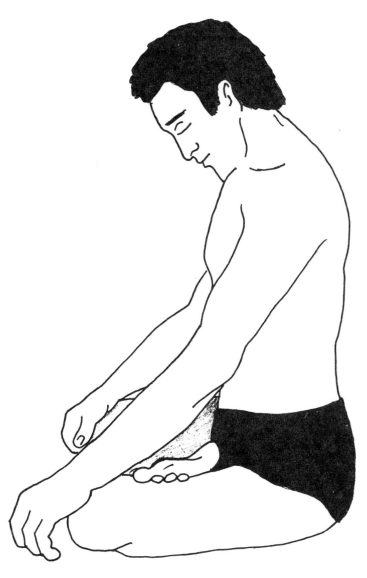

Jalandhara Bandha

It is said in *Sivasamhita* that by putting pressure on the carotid sinus nerves a blissful state of mind is experienced. In other words, when the chin lock is practiced, both in exhalation and inhalation, control of *vijnani nadi* becomes easy. But it takes a long time—sometimes years—for the yogi to have control of the *jalandhara bandha.*

When the chin lock is not applied after the retention of the breath, the air inhaled wants to rush out, after deep inhalation, even if the glottis is kept closed. So it rushes through the auditory tubes and disturbs, or brings about, various disorders in the inner ear. Therefore *jalandhara bandha* is applied to prevent such disorders. The glottis is first closed; then, by proper application of the chin lock, practicing *khumbhaka* becomes easy.*

Uddiyana Bandha—The Abdominal Lift:

Uddiyana is an exercise which involves the diaphragm, ribs and abdominal muscles, and it can be practiced either standing or sitting in one of the meditative postures. In the standing position the feet are approximately two feet apart. Keep the spine straight,

*A few doctors in India put pressure on the carotid arteries and thus give yogic anesthesia to the patient. They even perform minor surgery with this "anesthetic." The same principle has been adopted by martial art experts, especially in the school of Kung Fu. Children often experience that pleasant feeling of "passing out" when they unconsciously learn to put pressure on the carotid artery. Through *jalandhara bandha* yogis bring about conscious control of this phenomenon and thus attain a state of joy before doing meditation.

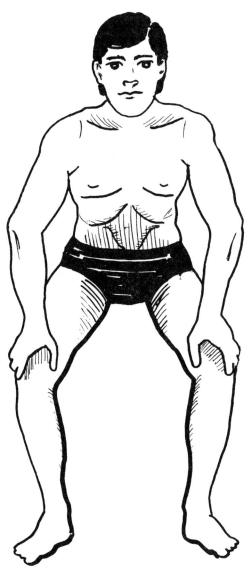

Uddiyana Bandha

bend the knees slightly and lean forward from the waist far enough to place the palms of the hands just above the knees. Exhale completely, and place the chin on the hollow of the throat. Without inhaling, suck the abdominal muscles in and up, pulling the navel toward the spine. This motion pulls the diaphragm up and creates a cavity on the front side of the abdomen under the rib cage. The back will curve slightly. This position is held for as long as it remains comfortable. Then slowly inhale and relax.

Never force the abdominal muscles outward; use force only in pulling the muscles in and upward. Do not practice this exercise if there is any problem with high blood pressure, hiatal hernia, ulcers or heart disorders. Women should not practice it during menstruation or pregnancy. *Uddiyana* is one of the finest exercises for all the abdominal organs.

Mulabandha:

Mulabandha, or the anus lock, is an exercise in which the sphincter muscles are contracted. Both the external muscles (anal sphincter) and the internal sphincter muscles are contracted and then held. This *bandha* is used during *pranayama* and meditation.

Mudras:

Mudras mean *to seal*. There are a number of *mudras* mentioned in the yoga texts including *maha mudra*, *khecari mudra*, *aswini mudra*, *yoga mudra*, *vajroli*, *jnana mudra, Vishnu mudra* and others.

A *mudra* used during meditation is *jnana mudra*. Once the student has arranged his feet and legs and has placed his body in a comfortable sitting posture, it is important that the arms, hands and fingers be arranged accordingly, so that they do not become a source of distraction. *Jnana mudra*, or the finger lock, is then applied. Although there are various ways of placing the fingers, the simplest is to place the thumb and the forefinger together and rest the hands, palms downward, on the knees. *Vishnu mudra*, which is used during *pranayama* exercises, is described in the *nadi shodhanam* section.

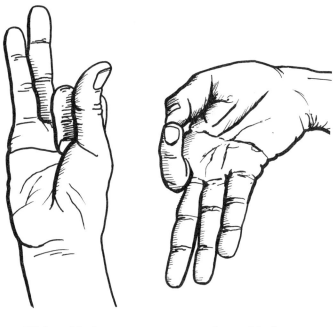

Vishnu Mudra   Jnana Mudra

The Importance of Breath Awareness in Meditation:
Breath awareness is an essential part of meditation. The most well-established schools teach breath awareness before leading a student toward advanced techniques of meditation, but some of the modern schools of meditation and relaxation do not understand its importance, and they cannot therefore lead their students to deeper states of meditation.

The mind is in the habit of identifying itself with the objects of the world, and it does not become aware of internal states as long as it remains in its dissipated condition. With systematic discipline, however, the mind starts traveling inward toward the more subtle, finer levels of consciousness, and when one attains a state of perfect stillness and tranquility, that which is beyond the mind reveals itself.

In learning to meditate, tranquility of the mind is an important factor, but even more important is breath awareness. The primary step is to find a steady, comfortable and easy posture. The second step is to develop calm, serene and even breathing. Third, a calm and steady mind is the only means for experiencing the deeper levels of being. The fourth step is control of the conscious mind, for this control can make one dynamic and creative. In the fifth step the involuntary system as well as a vast part of the unconscious mind, including the memory, is brought under conscious control, and in the sixth step the mind becomes aware that it is conditioned by time, space and causation. Through meditation, or constant awareness, the mind can be trained to remain aware of the now, which is an essential part of eternity. In the seventh step constant awareness is developed by the regular practice of meditation, and the highest state of *turiya* is attained. This state of mind is full of bliss, peace, happiness and wisdom.*

After serious observation and analysis of its functionings, yogis have found that the mind forms the habit of being conditioned, either by remembering past experiences or by imagining the future. There is no technique which helps it to become aware of the now except that of meditation and contemplation. But meditation is not a method of allowing the mind to roam aimlessly. It is a conscious effort of coordinating the body, the breath and the mind. In the monastic tradition teachers do not teach the advanced techniques of meditation unless they see the signs and symptoms of the stillness of the body and the serenity of the breath.

When a student learns to still his body he becomes aware of many tremors, twitching, and movements that he was not aware of before. Since childhood he has learned to move, but no one has taught him how to be still, and sitting still is very important, for the less movement there is in the body, the steadier the mind will be. All of the movements, gestures, tremors, and twitchings of the body are caused by an undisciplined and untrained mind, and when a student examines his behavior, he finds that not a single act or gesture is independent. The mind moves first, and then the body moves—and the more the

* For further details see Swami Ajaya, *Yoga Psychology* and also Usharbudh Arya, *Superconscious Meditation* (Honesdale, PA: The Himalayan Institute), 1978.

body moves, the more the mind dissipates. When the student has learned to be still, however, and begins learning the techniques of breath awareness and meditation, he becomes aware that he can have conscious control over his body, his breath and his mind.

So the first thing one must learn is to sit still. The right posture is one that makes one steady and comfortable, and it is one in which all or most of the body parts are free from the pressure of the other body parts.

Sukhasana, or Easy Posture:

Sitting with the head, neck and trunk straight, place the left foot beneath the right knee and the right foot beneath the left knee. Each knee rests on the opposite foot. Place the hands on the corresponding knees and apply the finger lock. This is a posture for beginners.

Swastikasana, or Auspicious Pose:

This posture was so named by the ancient Aryans. Here, the heels and ankle bones are not aligned. Bend the left leg at the knee and place the sole of the left foot against the right thigh. Place the right foot on top of the left calf, and put the outer edge of the foot and the toes between the thigh and calf muscles. The big toe should be visible. Pull the toes of the left foot between the right thigh and calf so that the big toe is visible. Place hands on the corresponding knees, joining the fingers in the finger lock.

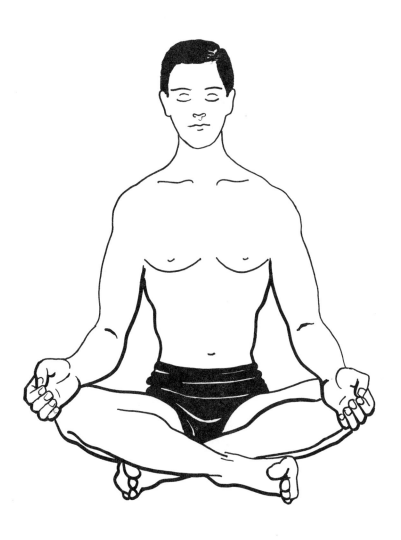

Sukhasana, or Easy Posture

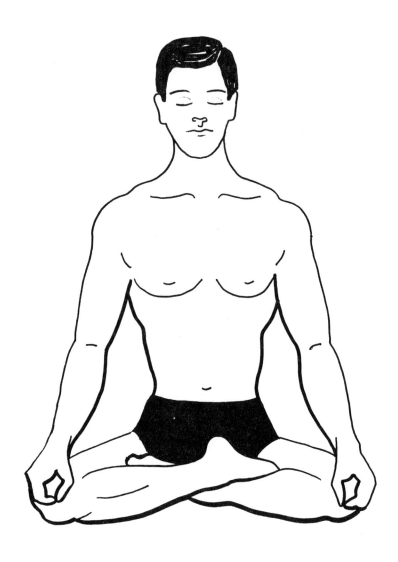

Swastikasana, or Auspicious Posture

Siddhasana, or Accomplished Pose:

A favorite of yogins, *siddhasana* is called the accomplished posture, or the posture of adepts. In it advanced yogis meditate for hours and hours together or practice advanced *pranayama* techniques. Place the left heel at the perineum and the right heel at the pubic bone above the organ of generation. Arrange the feet and legs so that the ankles are in one line or touch one another. Place the toes of the right foot between the left thigh and calf so that only the big toe is visible. Pull the toes of the left foot up between the right thigh and calf so the big toe is visible. This is the finest of all postures, but it could be uncomfortable for those who are not advanced.

Padmasana, or Lotus Posture:

Padma means lotus. It is a symbol of yoga because just as the lotus grows in the water but keeps its petals untouched by the water, so does the yogi live in the world and yet remain above. Immense benefits are derived from this posture. To do it one should take one's place firmly on a cushion (or a four-folded blanket or a pillow). Bend the left leg at the knee joint; turn up the sole and place the foot firmly at the right groin. Similarly, fold the right leg, turning up the sole and placing it firmly at the left groin. Both heels should press firmly against the abdominal wall. Place the hands on the corresponding knees and assume *jnana mudra* (the finger lock). To apply *bandhas* or locks in this posture is complicated, and without expert guidance they should not be applied. Applying *bandhas* in *padmasana* for a long time definitely

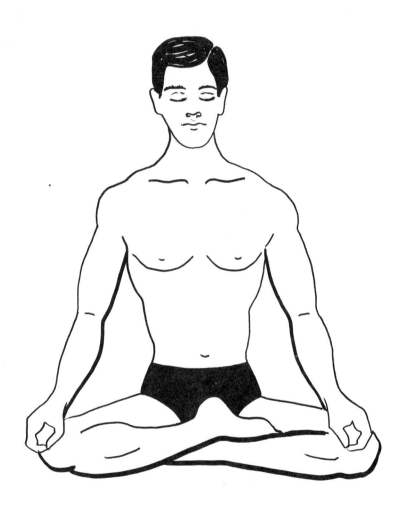

Siddhasana, or Accomplished Posture

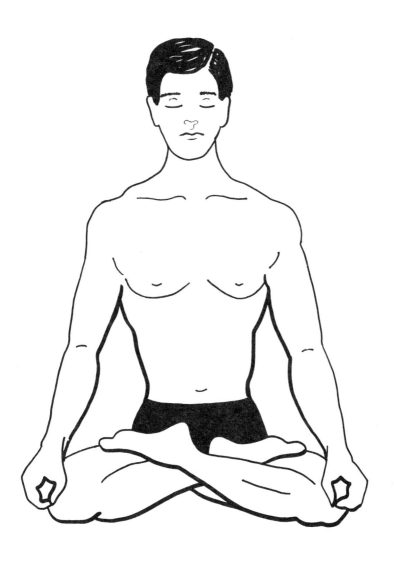

Padmasana, or Lotus Posture

disturbs the intestinal movement and creates gastric problems. As an exercise, however, it is one of the finest for abdominal muscles.

Maitriyasana:
For a modern man it is sometimes more convenient to sit on a straight-backed wooden chair, keeping the head, neck and trunk straight and placing the hands on his knees. The legs should not be crossed but firmly placed on the ground. Buddhist scriptures describe this posture.

Vajrasana, or Kneeling Posture:
Sit in a kneeling position with the head, neck and trunk straight. Place the hands, palms downward, above the knees. This posture is mostly practiced in non-yogic traditions like Zen and the Islamic tradition. It can also be used for meditation, but if it is continued for a long time it sometimes creates a problem of muscle pull by overstretching the ligaments of the foot.

Having found a comfortable, stable and easy posture, the student will then be able to become aware of his breath. Breath awareness is a reliable guide for experiencing the higher level of consciousness and for making the mind one-pointed, and it prepares the meditator for applying *sushumna* (a state of joyous mind which is the prerequisite for meditation). There are only

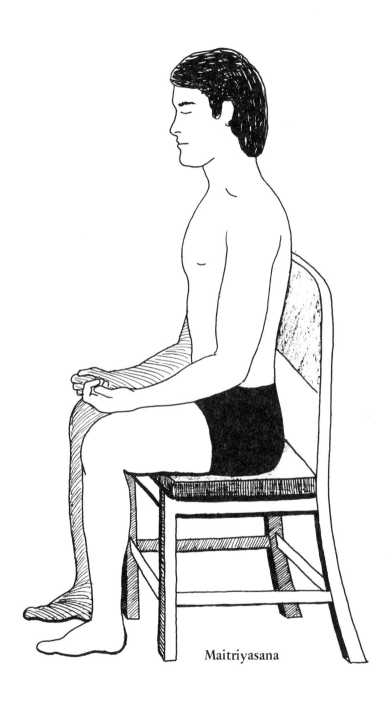

Maitriyasana

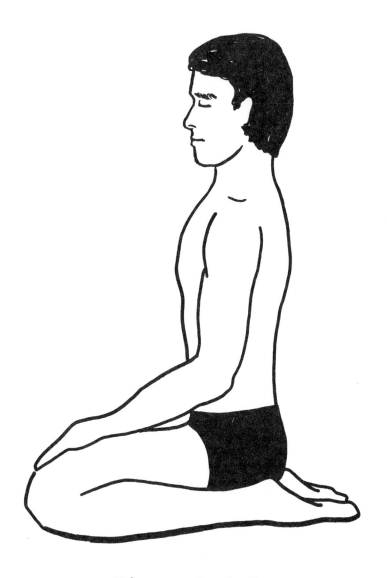

Vajrasana, or Kneeling Posture

two or three techniques for applying *sushumna:* 1) concentrating on the bridge between the two nostrils, 2) doing *pranayama* breathing exercises and applying *jalandhara bandha* and 3) meditating on the *chakra* system. In breath awareness the duration of inhalation and exhalation is carefully judged mentally, and the mind very closely and intimately follows the movement of the breath. Here lies the difference between breathing exercises and breath awareness. In breathing exercises one is taught to keep a count of the amount of air inhaled and exhaled, but in breath awareness it is done mentally only. No fingers are used to close the nostrils. Through breath awareness the power of attention is strengthened, and attention is the very key for meditation. In breath awareness there is no external distraction, and the attention is not dissipated.

So breath awareness is vital for a student who wants to learn the higher techniques of meditation. When he sits in a calm, quiet place in a comfortable, steady posture, and when body tremors do not become a source of disturbance, he becomes aware of four irregularities in his breath: shallowness of breath, jerks in the breath, sound in the breath, and a pause between inhalation and exhalation. We are not discussing breathing exercises here. Breath awareness is an advanced technique; it comes after one has practiced the various exercises of breathing described above. Some schools, like the Buddhist and Zen schools of meditation, do not teach these exercises as do the yoga schools. But for them also, breath awareness is the most important step in meditation.

The breath is a bridge, or link, between the body and the mind. Advanced yogis observe that the breath is like a thermometer which registers the conditions of the mind and the influence of the external environment on the body, and those who have studied breath behavior also know their mental and physical behavior. Their lives are guided by their control of *swaras*, or life ripples.

One's breath behavior can also warn one of illness. For example, when the body suffers from fever the nostrils start behaving in an unusual way. One of them, for instance, may either start flowing excessively or become blocked. In such a condition, naturally, the respiratory system does not function normally; the lungs, heart and related systems are disturbed, and in such a condition the mind loses its equilibrium. The advanced yogis use their breath behavior to watch the capacity of their minds and bodies, and they control the behavior of their breath by various exercises.

For the hathayogins *pranayama* is the final way of liberation; for the rajayogins *pranayama* is equally important. According to this school, after having attained a still and comfortable posture, breath awareness is an important step for awakening the *sushumna*. Although the word *sushumna* cannot be translated into English, according to me it means the state of mind that is undisturbed and joyous when the two nostrils are flowing evenly. When the breath starts flowing freely and smoothly through both nostrils the mind attains that state. Such a mental condition is necessary in order for the mind to travel into deeper levels of consciousness for if the mind is not brought to a state of joy, it cannot remain steady, and an unsteady mind is not at all fit for meditation. Another school, which teaches the awakening of *kundalini*, says that without awakening the *sushumna*, deep meditation and the awakening of the *kundalini* is impossible. The process of awakening the *sushumna* is possible only when a student starts enjoying being still. The moment he starts meditating on the flow of breath he starts observing the various defects in its flow—noise, shallowness and that which disturbs him the most, the pause between inhalation and exhalation. Much has been spoken about this in the scriptures, but practice makes one increasingly aware of its importance. When a student starts meditating on the flow of breath the pause distracts his mind. Some of the scriptures say that the pause can be expanded, some say that it can be omitted. In the beginning, however, one has to go through the exercises of *pranayama* and later the exercises of breath retention under the guidance of a competent teacher. Those who do not want to do *pranayama* exercises can still do meditation, but without breath awareness a deep state of meditation is impossible.

What should be the object of meditation? Various schools recommend different objects for making the mind one-pointed. These are both concrete and abstract; they can be sound syllables, *mantras*, images etc., but none of these objects is helpful in the long run without breath awareness.

The breath and the mind are interdependent. If one retains the breath, his mind starts becoming one-pointed; if the breath is irregular and jerky, the mind is dissipated. After attaining a steady posture, meditation on the breath, or breath awareness, is very natural. Breath awareness strengthens the mind and makes it easier for it to become inward. When the mind starts following the flow of the breath, one becomes aware of the reality that all the creatures of the world are breathing the same breath. There is a direct communication between the student and that center of the cosmos which supplies life breath to all living creatures. This is a living philosophy of life. As long as the center, or living unit in the human life, receives vital force, or *prana*, through the breath, the body-mind relationship is sustained. When this communication is disrupted the conscious mind fails and the body is separated from the inner unit of life. This separation is called death.

It is advisable for beginners to develop the habit of breath awareness and not to worry about any other kind of object for the mind to rest upon, for breath awareness is a most natural and essential step for attaining the higher state of meditation.

Meditation is the sustained state of one-pointedness of the mind. In deep meditation the one-pointed mind is able to pierce through the layers of the conscious and unconscious minds to the superconscious state, and this breakthrough is called *samadhi*. On achieving it, one is freed from all bondage and transcends the limitations of time, space and causation. The microcosm expands to become the macrocosm as a drop of water merges with the ocean and becomes the ocean. The individual *atman* is united with and achieves total identity with the cosmic *Brahman*. Such a one has found the kingdom of God within himself and has won the ultimate freedom—freedom from the endless chain of birth and death. The evolution of man to God is now complete.

Index

A

control of, 98

B

bandhas, 122
jalandhara, 122, 124, 139
mula, 126
in padmasana, 133, 136
uddiyana, 124, 126
bhastrika, 118-119
bhramari pranayama, 119-120
Brahman, 104, 142
brahmarandra, 100, 101
breath
and emotions, 105-106
irregularities, 139
patterns, 11-12, 19, 21, 52-53, 105-106
pause in, 141
and prana, 8-9, 11, 92-96
retention of, 95, 117-118, 121, 141
and yogic feats, 1
breath awareness, 17-22
and breathing exercises, difference between, 139
and meditation, 128-130, 136, 139-143
breathing, see also "diaphragmatic breathing," "inhalation," "breathing exercises"
abdominal muscles used in, 44-45
anatomy of, 34-39
and autonomic nervous system, 48-49, 50
chest, 39, 47-50, 109

emphysema, 31
emotions and breath, 105-106
energy
  flow of, and respiration, 11
  level of in man, 6
  and matter, relationship between, 7-8
  patterns of, in a leaf, 13-14
  patterns of, in man, 12
erectile tissue in nose, 76-77, 85, 86
evolution
  Western theory, 15
  yoga (Eastern) theory, 15-16

F

"fight or flight" response, 48, 49, 109
Fliess, Wilhelm, 76
Freud, 8, 76

G

gaj karni (upper wash), 75
God, kingdom of, 143

H

hatha yoga, 104, 122, 140
heart disease and breathing, 53-54

L

lacrimal glands, 71-72
laterality in nose, 76-80
libido, 8
limbic system, 87
lotus posture, 133, 136
Lowen, Alexander, and breathing, 47-48
lymphoid tissue, 70

M

maitriyasana, 136
makarasana, 112
manipura chakra, 101
manomaya kosha, 14
meditation, 4, 72-73
    and breath awareness, 128-130, 139-143
    object of, 141
    postures of, 130, 133, 136
    and *sushumna,* 100, 107
    teaching advanced techniques of, 129
menstrual cramps and nasal inflammation, 77
mind
    and breath, 140-143
    and energy, 14, 91-92
    and meditation, 128-130
mind/body problem
    breath as link, 140-143
    Eastern approach to, 4-6, 8-11, 13-15, 105, 129

R

raja yoga, 104, 140
relaxation and breathing, 41
respiration, see also, "breath," "breathing," 28-31
diseases of, 31-33
rhinologists, 59-60, 84, 85

S

samadhi, 104, 142
sandbag breathing, 112-113
sandhya, 100
sahasrara chakra, 101, 104
samana, 92-93
sexual activity and nose, 76
shakti, 104
shavasana, 110, 112
shiva, 104
siddhasana, 133
sinus headache, 71
sinuses, 70-71
sinusitis, 70-71
sitali pranayama, 120
sitkari pranayama, 120
Sivasamhita, 124
sleep apnea, 52-54
soul, individual and cosmic, 104
sukhasana, 130
surfactant in alveoli, 42

suryabhedana pranayama, 120
sushumna, 100-104, 106-107
    methods for applying, 136, 139, 140
sutra neti, 108
swadhisthana chakra, 101
swastikasana, 130
swara yogis, 78-79
swaras, 140
sympathetic nervous system, 49, 50, 96

T

tonsil, 70
turbinates, 64-65, 77, 86, 106, 107
    removal of, 85
turiya, 129

U

udana, 92
uddiyana bandha, 124-126
ujjayi pranayama, 119
Upanishads
    and levels of existence, 8
    and pranic level of being, 10, 14
upper wash, 75

V

vagus nerve, 96, 97

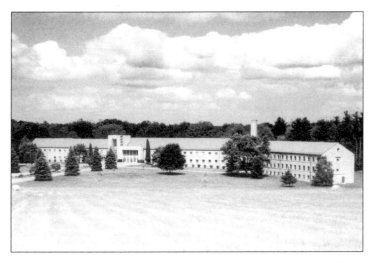

The main building of the national headquarters, Honesdale, Pa.

THE HIMALAYAN INSTITUTE

SINCE ITS ESTABLISHMENT IN 1971, the Himalayan Institute has been dedicated to helping people grow physically, mentally, and spiritually by combining the best knowledge of both the East and the West. Institute programs emphasize holistic health, yoga, and meditation, but the Institute is much more than its programs.

Our national headquarters is located on a beautiful 400-acre campus in the rolling hills of the Pocono Mountains of north-eastern Pennsylvania. The atmosphere here is one to foster growth, increased inner awareness, and calm. Our grounds provide a wonderfully peaceful and healthy setting for our seminars and extended programs. Students from around the world join us here to attend programs in such diverse areas as hatha yoga, meditation, stress reduction, Ayurveda, nutrition, Eastern philosophy, psychology, and other subjects. Whether the programs are for weekend meditation retreats, week-long seminars on spirituality, months-long residential programs, or holistic health services, the attempt here is to provide an environment of gentle inner progress. We invite you to join with us in the ongoing process of personal growth and development.

The Institute is a nonprofit organization. Your membership in the Institute helps to support its programs. Please call or write for information on becoming a member.

Institute Programs, Services, and Facilities

All Institute programs share an emphasis on conscious, holistic living and personal self-development. You may enjoy any of a number of diverse programs, including:

Special weekend or extended seminars to teach skills and techniques for increasing your ability to be healthy and enjoy life

Holistic health services

Meditation retreats and advanced meditation instruction

Vegetarian cooking and nutritional training

Hatha yoga and exercise workshops

Residential programs for self-development

The Institute publishes a free *Quarterly Guide to Programs and Other Offerings*. To request a copy, or for further information, call 800-822-4547, fax 717-253-9078, e-mail himalaya@epix.net, or write the Himalayan Institute/RR 1, Box 400/Honesdale, PA 18431.

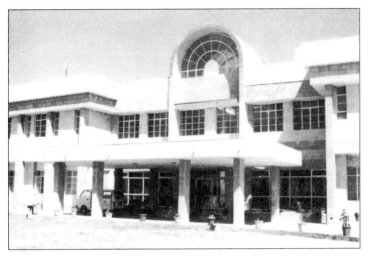

The main building of the hospital, outside Dehra Dun

The Himalayan Institute Charitable Hospital

A major aspect of the Institute's work around the world is its construction and management of a modern, comprehensive hospital and holistic health facility in the mountain area of Dehra Dun, India. Outpatient facilities are already providing medical care to those in need, and mobile units have been equipped to visit outlying villages. Constructions work on the main hospital building is progressing quickly.

We welcome financial support to help with the construction and the provision of services. We also welcome donations of medical supplies, equipment, or professinal expertise. If you would like further information on the hospital, please contact our headquarters in Honesdale, Pa.

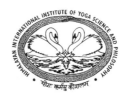

The Himalayan Institute Press

The Himalayan Institute Press has long been regarded as "The Resource for Holistic Living." We publish dozens of titles, as well as audio and video tapes, that offer practical methods for harmonious living and inner balance. Our approach addresses the whole person—body, mind, and spirit—integrating the latest scientific knowledge with ancient healing and self-development techniques.

As such, we offer a wide array of titles on physical and psychological health and well-being, spiritual growth through meditation and other yogic practices, and the means to stay inspired through reading sacred scriptures and ancient philosophical teachings.

Our health sidelines include The Neti™ Pot, the ideal tool for sinus and allergy sufferers, and The Breath Pillow,™ a unique tool for learning health-supportive breathing—the diaphragmatic breath.

Our bimonthly magazine, *Yoga International,* offers thought-provoking articles on all aspects of meditation and yoga, including yoga's sister science, Ayurveda.

Call 800-822-4547 for a free catalog.